You Can Beat Arthritis

A message of hope for the millions of sufferers
from arthritis, rheumatism and chronic back pain

by

Jeremy Michaels

IMPERIA BOOKS LIMITED

First published 1992
by Imperia Books Ltd.
© 1992 Imperia Books Ltd.

British Library Cataloguing
in Publication Data
A catalogue record for this book
is available from the British Library

ISBN 1 897656 01 7

Typeset by Carter Wordsmiths, London
Cover by The Green Street Press, Chelmsford

Published by
IMPERIA BOOKS LIMITED
Canada House, Blackburn Road, London NW6 1RZ
Printed in Great Britain by Black Bear Press Ltd. of Cambridge

Foreword by Dr. Ann Robinson

This is an excellent book – and much overdue. I have searched long and hard for a comprehensive yet comprehensible book about arthritis and I think this is as close as possible to that ideal.

There is one thing a seventy year old man with a painful arthritic hip and a young musician with rheumatoid arthritis of her hands have in common – that is a thirst for information. They need to know what is likely to happen to them, what conventional treatment is available from doctors and how they can help themselves to stave off disability.

And there is a burgeoning array of complementary or alternative therapies, all making extravagant claims, with extravagant fees to match. How does a person with arthritis find objective information about what the different therapies involve and which are the most valid?

The fact that so many arthritic sufferers turn to complementary therapies is testament to the fact that conventional medicine has failed them to a certain extent. It's not just that there are no absolute cures yet and that all drugs have some side effects. The problem remains that doctors don't have the time necessary to explain all aspects of the disease and answer all the questions you want to ask.

As a GP, I am grateful to Jeremy Michaels for coming up with such a thorough review of arthritis in all its forms. There cannot be a family in Britain which does not have to confront these vexing conditions. This book should have a place on the bookshelf in every home.

Ann Robinson
M.B. B.S. D.C.H. D.R.C.O.G. M.R.C.G.P.

Contents

Oh, deep in my heart
I do believe
We shall overcome some day

- Zilphia Horton,
Pete Seeger and others

Preface

The very mention of the words *arthritis* or *rheumatism* strikes fear into many people. It conjures up the prospect of a lifetime racked with pain – a vision of people with pitifully distorted limbs, confined to wheelchairs. Despair deepens when it is realised that the basic causes are unknown to medical science and that no certain cure has yet been discovered.

A very large number of people suffer from one or other of the many illnesses included under the general description *arthritis, rheumatism* or *chronic back pain*. It is estimated that, in the United Kingdom alone, well over eight million people consult their doctors about them every year.

Though more common among the elderly, arthritis is certainly not a disease of old age. Persons of all ages – men, women and children – can be and are affected. Over one million people under forty-five have arthritis, including some twelve thousand children.

The terms *arthritis* and *rheumatism* cover a huge range of related ailments. Arthritis is used to describe those involving trouble with the joints alone; and rheumatism is the umbrella term used to describe those also involving the muscles and other soft tissues. Attacks vary between mild episodes, which disappear after a time, to severe illness that can lead to crippling disability. The good news is that, with modern treatment, comparatively few cases need result in serious disablement.

This book's primary purpose is to bring a message of hope to sufferers. They need no longer resign themselves passively to a life of pain and restriction. They should not just sit back and accept arthritis as inevitable; for there are many choices of both conventional and alternative therapies now available – and one or more of them may well bring relief. Nor should sufferers delay an attempt to deal with their condition until their joints become irreversibly damaged.

Though complete cures may perhaps be unusual, the illness *can* be mastered, its effects minimised and an acceptable quality of life maintained. The biggest enemies of people with rheumatic disease are ignorance, despair and resignation.

Overcoming arthritis certainly requires the help of doctors, therapists and other experts. But the patient's attitude is an essential part of the process. There can be no substitute for his or her own active and informed participation – first in coming to terms with, and then eventually in mastering, the worst aspects of the condition.

Though intelligent self-help is an essential part of learning to cope, it must be stressed that a *do it yourself* attitude is not recommended. For the vast majority, it is dangerous to proceed without sound medical guidance.

This book attempts first to explain simply, in non-technical language, the many different forms rheumatic disease can take.

A large range of available treatments is then outlined, ranging from conventional medical methods to the wide variety of *alternative* or *complementary* therapies claimed to have helped many thousands of sufferers.

The book's purpose is to inform – not to make judgements. Adopting a commonsense approach, it aims to set out what is involved, to survey the advice given and the claims made, and then to list what help and support is available and where fuller information can be found. Some personal comments, arising from the author's own feelings during and after the writing of the book, are included in the Epilogue.

The contents of this volume are not original. On the contrary, its text has been influenced by several excellent publications dealing with the various topics. Acknowledgement of these sources is included by way of books recommended for further reading. What may be unusual, though, is the presentation in one place of so many different approaches to the problems posed by rheumatic disease.

As parts of this book may be read separately from the rest, some advice and information has had to be repeated in different sections.

The struggle to prevent rheumatic disease from ruining the quality of a sufferer's life is very much worthwhile. Quoting the poet Dylan Thomas, though in slightly different context:

Do not go gentle into that good night.
Rage, rage against the dying of the light.

It is hoped that this volume will provide many readers with a useful guide to that struggle. May their efforts be crowned with success.

Part One

Introduction

The Human Body and Rheumatic Disease

How the Body Moves

The structure of the human body is its framework of bones – its skeleton, which gives the body its basic shape.

Muscles are elastic tissues attached at their leading ends to the bones by fibrous cords called *tendons*. The shortening and the lengthening of the different muscles fixed to a bone cause that bone to move; and most body movement is brought about that way.

A *joint* is the place where two bones meet and move relative to each other – elbows, ankles, knees, hips, etc.

The surfaces of the ends of bones, where they rub together at a joint, are capped with a smooth gristle-like substance called *cartilage*.

Bones are held in position at a joint by *ligaments*. These bind the joint together and act rather like broad elastic bands. The ligaments, together with other tissues, form a tough protective capsule which surrounds and encloses the entire joint.

On the inside of the capsule, closest to the joint itself, is a special membrane called the *synovial membrane* or the *synovium*. This produces a powerful lubricating fluid which fills the joint space to assist movement. It also nourishes the cartilage which has no blood supply of its own.

The rather more complex arrangement of joints between the bones of the spine, the vertebrae, are described in Part Two of this book.

The *bursa* is a small sac of fluid, often situated between a joint and the skin. Its purpose is to ease the movement of the skin or of a tendon over the hard, bony projection at a joint.

What Is Rheumatic Disease ?

In general, inflammation or trouble with one or more joints is known as *arthritis*. If the softer tissues such as muscles are also involved, the malady is called *rheumatism*. There are over two hundred different types of ailment in these main categories, and each has its own special name.

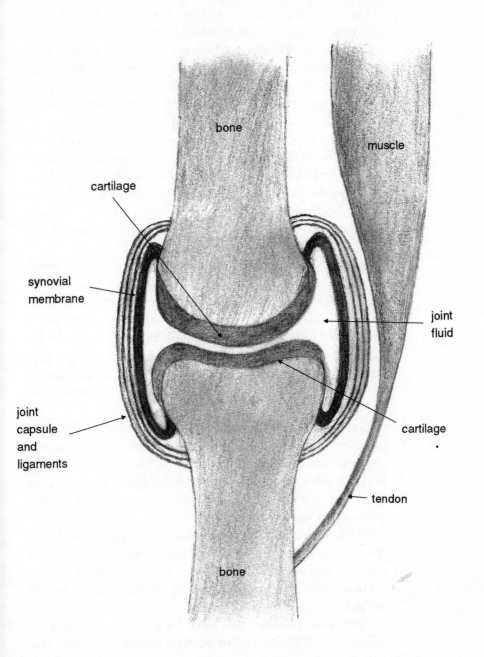

FIG. 1   A TYPICAL JOINT

The technical names used by doctors to describe the different conditions can themselves be intimidating at first sight to those without medical knowledge. But the general reader should remember that a name, however complicated, is just a name. Even the longest of them will soon become familiar – and especially if it is that of the particular complaint in which he or she is most interested.

Osteoarthritis (or osteoarthrosis, as it is sometimes called) is the commonest condition of all, affecting most people to some extent as they grow older. It is caused by wear and tear of the joints, particularly those larger joints which carry most of the body weight. It starts with damage to the cartilage lining of the ends of the bones where they rub together at a joint; and it can later affect the bones themselves.

Rheumatoid arthritis is a more acute ailment from which over a million people may be suffering at any one time. In this condition, the membrane lining the joint (the synovium) becomes inflamed and releases substances (enzymes) which then attack other parts of the joint. Typically, a person has acute flare-ups which eventually subside – but during which, apart from the pain and inflammation, a sufferer often feels ill for long periods and experiences symptoms not unlike those of influenza.

Backache is usually a debilitating though temporary problem caused by mechanical strain to the muscles or ligaments attached to the spine. It can be brought on by lifting heavy weights or by making sudden, awkward movements. With rest and care, these conditions often heal themselves after a short time.

Of the arthritic disorders causing back pain, ankylosing spondylitis, spondylosis and disc problems (such as *slipped disc*) are among the most serious. Back pain for which no certain cause can be identified is also included in this category.

Other joint pain can be caused by excess acid – gout; by infections – T.B., viruses or Reiter's disease; by widespread inflammation of body tissues – ankylosing spondylitis, S.L.E.

or P.M.R.; by weak bones – osteoporosis; and by degenerative diseases – spondylosis and disc problems.

The various soft-tissue rheumatic ailments, such as tennis elbow, golfer's elbow, frozen shoulder, housemaid's knee, fibrositis, bursitis and growing pains are localised and have shorter duration. They usually present less intractable problems and will be mentioned only briefly below.

The two complaints that between them affect millions of people – osteoarthritis and rheumatoid arthritis – are described first in Part Two of the book. Shorter accounts of the other rather less common conditions follow.

Conventional and Alternative Approaches

Diagnosis

It must be emphasised from the start that there is no viable alternative to skilled medical advice.

A doctor must be consulted if pains in muscles or joints persist for any length of time. Specialist advice should also be sought, promptly and without hesitation, in cases of further doubt.

The basis for all rational treatment must be sound diagnosis. Only after that can a safe course of action be planned. This applies equally to treatment by one of the alternative therapies, by more conventional medical means, or by a combination of both.

A whole battery of devices, including blood tests and X-rays is available for accurate diagnosis; and the main rheumatic and arthritic conditions can now be identified with confidence.

Rheumatic disease, as the entire range of conditions is called, is no longer accepted as inevitable or incurable by enlightened members of the medical profession. However, a great deal more research is needed before the actual causes of arthritis are understood and cures for it discovered.

The Latest Research

Conventional medical research is proceeding on these vital matters, much of it funded by private charities. The results so far are encouraging; and those engaged in the work hope that it will be possible to achieve more useful progress before long.

Another potentially valuable avenue of research is into food and environmental sensitivity, described in Part Five of this book. So far, only a limited number of clinical trials have been undertaken.

Research into most alternative therapies proceeds very slowly indeed, if at all. Funding for this work is scarce.

Medical and Surgical Treatment

Medical Treatment

Conventional medical treatment employs drugs to control peaks of illness. Symptoms are then eased by a combination of painkillers, sensible diet, physiotherapy and a proper balance between rest and exercise.

Several programmes, devised in conjunction with self-help groups, exist to guide sufferers in coming to terms with their condition and adjusting their patterns of everyday living to suit.

Rheumatology outpatient clinics at many hospitals have multi-disciplinary teams of experts which can offer a comprehensive physical and psychological approach to the problems of living with arthritis. The better ones are of special value for they seek to mobilise all the sufferer's own personal resources in an attempt to overcome the condition. Furthermore, they also tackle head-on the associated anxiety, stress and depression that so often accompany and aggravate the symptoms of rheumatic disease. Patients are referred to such clinics by their family doctor.

Surgical Treatment

Surgery is being used with increasing success to alleviate extreme conditions. This can involve simple repairs, the actual re-aligning of bones at a joint and even the removal and re-shaping of the ends of bones themselves.

In recent years, for example, the lives of thousands of patients with osteoarthritis of the hip have been transformed by operations to replace the defective joint with a new artificial joint made from metal and plastic. This has now become a standard surgical procedure.

Drugs

Drugs have two main functions, which are to control symptoms and to slow or modify the progress of the disease.

Though very useful to clear infection and reduce acute inflammation and pain, drugs often produce side-effects when used for prolonged periods. There is, as yet, no completely safe drug for arthritis. This problem will be discussed in detail in Part Three of this book.

Medical Attitudes to Alternative Therapies

Prince Charles and the B.M.A.

Prince Charles, when elected president of the British Medical Association in 1983, urged doctors to open their minds to:

> ... long neglected complementary methods of medicine which in the right hands can bring considerable relief, if not hope, to an increasing number of people.

However the final report, issued after the three-year long inquiry launched as the result of the Prince's comment, gave only limited recognition to the value of acupuncture and hypnotherapy for pain relief and to aspects of osteopathic and chiropractic manipulation. Most other therapies were dismissed out of hand both as unscientific and as unproven in their effectiveness.

Significantly though, the report did recognise as ideal the holistic principles espoused by the alternative therapists – in which it is the whole individual, body and mind, that is treated and not just the symptoms of a particular ailment.

The eminent doctors who compiled the report noted with regret that a doctor spends on average only one-eighth of the time on each patient as that expended by an alternative therapist. They remarked on the close relationship of confidence and trust so often developed between patient and therapist during the course of treatment and commented that this helped to establish a state of mind in which self-healing is most likely to occur.

The implication seems to be a grudging acceptance of some of the claims of alternative therapy – though on the basis of natural self-healing rather than on the contents of the actual therapy. Also, that conventional medicine could achieve similar results if only given the same amount of time for diagnosis and treatment.

The Conventional View

Though the situation is changing fast, and fewer doctors now dismiss all alternative therapies as *quack* remedies, the medical profession as a whole remains suspicious of non-conventional approaches.

Claims are made that alternative remedies often fail to prove themselves when subjected to controlled clinical trials. Sometimes one trial is said to have produced a positive result whilst parallel ones did not.

All that can be concluded safely is that, from a strictly scientific point of view, the value of most alternative therapies is not proven. It is always possible, of course, that this may be because of the very few trials that have actually been attempted, because of the inadequacy of the trials themselves or because some therapies are just not amenable to such methods of testing – but such speculation is beyond the scope of this book.

The most that many doctors will admit is that alternative therapies may sometimes bring temporary relief without the use of drugs.

They point out that illnesses often go into remission at some stage and that some are cured eventually by the body's natural processes without outside intervention. That factor, they say, may underpin belief in the efficacy of alternative therapies. In other words, it is the coincidental working of nature, rather than alternative therapy, that is responsible for many reported successes.

Others maintain that it is the patient's confidence that produces the result. In other words, mind over matter, a type of faith healing.

Most modern doctors, therefore, will not actively obstruct their patients in trying out alternative remedies for themselves. They reason that such remedies can do little harm and may even make the sufferers feel better by bringing them new sources of hope.

The Opinion of One Doctor

There is probably no such thing as a typical doctor; but a young, intelligent and progressive general practitioner, with a busy London practice, was asked for her detailed views on what she preferred to call complementary therapy. The following is a summary of what the doctor had to say.

The doctor first warned how essential it is to seek expert conventional medical guidance before embarking on courses of complementary therapy. Several features of back pain, for example, may be indications of serious conditions like bone tumours, breast or lung cancer with spread to the bone, a bone infection or ankylosing spondylitis. Signs to watch for in particular are constant or progressive pain, worse symptoms on resting at night, morning pain and stiffness, diffuse pain and tenderness, abdominal and gynaecological symptoms.

The conventional doctor's verdict on various alternative therapies was as follows.

Naturopathy. The underlying theory remains unproven even though some of the dietary guidelines are compatible with orthodox views on what constitutes a healthy diet. Further, there is no evidence that the diet of sufferers from arthritis is any worse than that of those not so afflicted. Fasting may be positively harmful if it leads to undernourishment. The doctor much resented what she saw as the arrogance of some naturopaths in their certainty that their theory and methods are correct.

Acupuncture. This can be effective in the relief of pain in many cases and is offered by some NHS pain clinics. Evidence that cures can be accomplished by this method is lacking.

Homeopathy. Homeopathic remedies can now be prescribed on the NHS. Medical opinion is generally much less

9

antagonistic to homeopathy. Many GPs are learning about it and employing some remedies as an adjunct to conventional treatment. The doctor was sceptical about the efficacy of the dilutions used, other than as a placebo.

Herbalism, Aromatherapy and Bach Therapy. Many conventional drugs derive from plants and herbs and there is some medical interest in their use. A Chinese herbal remedy for eczema has completed medical trials and is now prescribable on the NHS. If herbs are inactive, they do no good. If they contain active ingredients, they need critical assessment before use. Untested drugs are dangerous; and untested herbs are also best avoided.

Mind Therapies. Any therapy that relieves anxiety, stress or pain must be of value.

Osteopathy and Chiropractic. Practitioners undergo stringent training before they can qualify and register. Their knowledge of the anatomy of the back surpasses that of many doctors. Chiropractic has been compared favourably with other methods of treating back pain in several clinical trials. However, expert medical advice should always be sought before any manipulation of the neck is attempted.

Massage and Rolfing. These are useful between attacks of arthritis to encourage mobilisation and a feeling of wellbeing. Care is needed in the presence of vulnerable, inflamed joints.

Alexander Technique and Feldenkrais. These encourage good posture, may be beneficial and can do no harm.

Food Sensitivity. Allergies and arthritis are both very common in developed countries, but evidence that one causes the other is lacking. Excluding foods from the diet, one at a time, is unlikely to be harmful. But exclusion diets and faddish eating may be dangerous unless undertaken under expert nutritional guidance.

Alternative Therapies

Some alternative therapies aim to do more than just alleviate symptoms – and actually to *cure* arthritis. Though it is seldom claimed that badly damaged joints can be regenerated, it is hoped that any further deterioration may be arrested.

Naturopathy Allergy and Nutrition

Of the many treatments available, those based on the allergic properties of everyday foods, and those based on naturopathic treatment of the whole body, are perhaps the most important. The theory is that they start by ridding the patient of poisons accumulated by drugs and unsuitable food, and then aim to let the body's own natural defences take over to defeat the illness.

Homeopathy and Herbalism

Homeopathy, herbal therapy and traditional Chinese medicine (including acupuncture) have similar fundamental concepts of the natural self-healing power of the whole human being, body and mind.

Physical Intervention

Other systems and techniques are based on direct physical intervention or manipulation. These include massage and rolfing, osteopathy, chiropractic, acupuncture, reflexology, Alexander technique and Feldenkrais. Some aim to tackle a part of the basic cause of rheumatic disease. Others restrict themselves to easing the worst symptoms of the disease and thus enabling sufferers to live with far less pain and disability.

Mind Therapies

Different therapies concentrate more on the mental or emotional state of the patient. These include yoga, meditation and relaxation, parapsychology, biofeedback and different forms of metaphysical healing.

Other Therapies

The advocates of many more methods, too numerous to list in full here, also claim that these can help in tackling rheumatic disease. They range from Bach Flower therapy to aromatherapy, Tai Chi and the wearing of copper bracelets.

Dietary supplements – such as bee venom, cider vinegar, extracts from New Zealand green-lipped mussels and extracts from deep-water sharks – are also said to relieve bad symptoms. Some of these products have been used as the basis for cures.

Combinations Different courses of treatment may be devised, utilising several of the above techniques at the same time. They avoid the use of drugs and attempt to treat the whole body and mind by natural methods.

Claims A very large number of people claim to have derived benefit from alternative therapies – sometimes moderate relief and sometimes dramatic improvement or even complete cure.

To such people, the lack of a convincing scientific explanation for the result of their therapy matters little. It is the result that is all-important. Medical science can discover reasons for it later.

Common Ground

There is more common ground than is often supposed between enlightened conventional and non-conventional methods of managing rheumatic disease; and it is hard to avoid the conclusion that alternative, or complementary, therapies are having an influence on more orthodox medical practice.

Diagnosis As mentioned above, proper diagnosis is an essential precondition of all treatment. So too is the positive interest and participation of the patient in all aspects of the programme.

Stress The conquest of anxiety, stress and depression, by whatever means, is another vital ingredient – though the use of drugs for this or any other purpose is strongly discouraged in alternative therapies.

Diet Sensible diet to promote physical well-being is common to all treatments.

Exercise and Rest Many exercise techniques, and specialised help from experts such as occupational therapists, are equally at home in both schools.

Manipulative therapy is also a common feature of much conventional and alternative management. Though the underlying ideologies may differ, there is often little difference in what actually is done.

Combined Approach

It certainly need not be either one thing or the other, conventional medicine or alternative therapy. In fact a truly common sense approach may well employ the best of all available treatments.

Drugs and conventional medicine may be used first to conquer infection and subdue acute pain and inflammation. A gradualist plan can then be adopted, trying whichever combination of alternative therapies is thought best suited to the particular condition; and then proceeding patiently on the basis of trial and error.

Part Two

The Diseases

General

This part of the book, which describe the symptoms of rheumatic disease in more detail, may make for rather depressing reading.

There is little mention in it of the very positive measures that can be taken to mitigate most aspects of the conditions, all of which are described in Parts Three, Four and Five of the book.

The reader may prefer to skip this section at first, returning to it later when a better idea has been obtained of what medical and alternative therapies have to offer.

Osteoarthritis (or Osteoarthrosis)

What Is It?

The ends of two bones, where they rub together in movement at a joint, are each lined with a smooth gristle-like substance called *Cartilage*. These cartilage linings, lubricated by a special fluid, provide smooth and slippery contact surfaces for the bones; and that helps them move easily against each other when required.

Thinning and roughening of the cartilage linings in a joint is the first sign of osteoarthritis. As the condition progresses, the cartilage flakes and splits, and may even disappear altogether, leaving the bone ends to rub directly against each other. The bones then react against this unaccustomed rough treatment, causing more trouble, pain and disability.

Osteoarthritis, therefore, is not really a disease but rather a local condition caused by the wearing and breakdown of the cartilage. It can affect several joints in the body or just a single joint.

The loss of the cartilage in a joint can clearly be seen on X-ray photographs often used to diagnose osteoarthritis.

Who Is Affected ...

Osteoarthritis can attack young people; but more usually is a condition associated with advancing age. For that reason some people, including doctors, accept its onset as inevitable

... and What Joints Are Most At Risk?

and remain passive in its wake. Feelings of hopelessness and even depression often follow such dismissive diagnosis and inhibit the robust attitude needed to combat its effects.

Indeed, the joints of most people over sixty will reveal some sign of osteoarthritis when examined by X-ray. However the body seems to cope naturally with slight deterioration, adjusting and healing itself; and so no pain or other symptoms are noticed by the majority of those affected.

Osteoarthritis affects slightly more women than men; and can often start after the menopause. Women suffer particularly from arthritis of the joints of the fingers and thumbs where bony knobs are formed, as well as from arthritis of the knees. Men and women are equally troubled by arthritis of the hips, the lower back, the neck and the big toe. Other joints too can become arthritic, especially those previously damaged by accident or by surgery.

What Actually Happens?

As the cartilage lining to the bone ends wears, the bones themselves become subjected to unusual stress as they grate together in movement. Parts of the joint become irritated and change in an attempt to adjust to the new conditions.

The bone ends thicken and distort. They grow bony lumps along their edges in an effort to relieve the pressure. The amount of joint fluid increases in volume, causing swelling. The joint sometimes, but not always, becomes slightly inflamed.

Movement of such joints becomes progressively more difficult, causing stress, distortion and pain every time they are forced. Thus a cycle of successive waves of pain, followed by further damage, is established.

In time, with constant exercise, the bone ends themselves sometimes wear smooth, thus allowing freer movement with less discomfort.

Osteoarthritis of the spine does not usually cause symptoms unless there is pressure on a nerve. The various back conditions such as ankylosing spondilitis, spondylosis and slipped disc are all discussed separately in the next chapter.

What Are The First Signs?

The joints stiffen and become painful, especially first thing in the morning and after exercise when one is tired. Movement becomes restricted and cracking noises are heard. A little swelling may also be noticeable.

How Does It Develop?

The symptoms gradually increase with time but not continuously. Bad periods alternate with easier spells.

In a few cases, the condition improves and then almost disappears. In most others it reaches its peak after several years and then becomes less acute. For an unfortunate minority, the arthritis becomes increasingly painful and in time leads to the total disablement of the affected joint.

What is the Conventional Medical Treatment?

It must be remembered that conventional medicine has not yet discovered the cause or a cure for osteoarthritis.

Prevention, by means of health education, is playing an increasingly important part in the struggle against the condition. Keeping the weight down, keeping mobile and avoiding strain to the joints are the keys to preventing, or at least delaying, the onset of osteoarthritis.

Symptoms may be relieved by the use of standard pain-killing drugs such as paracetamol or aspirin. Slight inflammation can also to some extent be suppressed by drugs, which can sometimes be injected into the joint itself. The use of drugs is discussed in Part Three of this book.

Conventional therapy, designed to overcome the worst effects of all kinds of arthritis and maintain a good quality of life for the sufferer, is described in Part Three.

Surgery, such as hip replacement operations, which now bring new hope to people with crippled joints, is also described later.

Rheumatoid Arthritis

What Is It?

Rheumatoid arthritis is a mysterious inflammatory disease of the joints. It often persists for long periods and can result in permanent injury.

Inflammation is usually a part of the body's healing processes. The supply of blood and other fluids to a damaged part increases, causing the swelling and sensations of heat and pain known as inflammation. This normally tends to isolate the injury, helps to overcome infection and aids recovery.

For some unknown reason, rheumatoid arthritis causes this natural process to reverse. Instead of promoting healing, the inflammation actually does harm.

The capsule of tissues surrounding and enclosing a joint is lined with a membrane called the *Synovium*. This produces a special fluid which normally lubricates and nourishes the smooth cartilage lining to the ends of the bones where they rub together in movement.

In rheumatoid arthritis, the synovium becomes inflamed and remains so for a long time. The resulting fluid attacks and eventually destroys the different parts of the joint.

Laboratory tests of samples of blood and joint fluid are often used to help diagnose the disease in its early stages. Later joint damage can then be tracked by X-ray.

Who Is Affected and What Joints Are Most At Risk?

Rheumatoid arthritis affects three times more women than men. It can begin at any age, including childhood, but more usually first appears in middle life.

Wrists and knuckles are almost always first affected. The balls of the feet and the knees are also likely candidates. But the disease can strike anywhere and at several joints at the same time.

A distinctive feature of rheumatoid arthritis, as opposed to osteoarthritis, is that it often attacks corresponding joints on each side of the body simultaneously.

What Happens?

Due to causes as yet unknown, the synovial membrane becomes inflamed and remains so for long periods, before subsiding for a time and flaring up again.

19

Cells from the inflamed membrane divide and grow, entering into the fluid that lubricates the joint. There is also an increased supply of blood to the joint.

The extra blood, together with the inflammatory cells, cause the joint to swell and feel warm to the touch. It stiffens and becomes painful.

The cells also release complex substances called enzymes into the joint. These in turn cause further irritation; and the cycle continues.

Eventually, unless checked, the enzymes damage the smooth cartilage lining to the ends of the bones. They also attack the surrounding capsule of tissues and the tendons. After some years they even eat away the corners of the bones themselves. The joint deforms and becomes incapable of much movement.

The active and acute phases of the disease are often accompanied by pain, weakness, general aching and fatigue, even a slight fever - in fact rather like the symptoms of influenza. Lumps (nodules) can appear beneath the skin in places like the elbows.

Unlike osteoarthritis, which affects several joints only, rheumatoid arthritis is a disease of the entire body. Therefore symptoms occasionally occur in other places outside the joints, such as the lungs and the eyes. Anaemia is another not unusual consequence.

What Are The First Signs?

The disease usually makes a gradual start, with vague muscular pains and a general feeling of tiredness and irritability.

Problems with the joints follow soon afterwards. Those of the wrist, fingers and balls of the feet are often the first to be affected. They swell and become stiff, especially first thing in the morning; but the discomfort wears off with exercise during the day.

How Does It Develop?

This is a very complicated disease and it affects different people in many different ways. Doctors are rarely able to predict the outcome for any one patient.

It is important to stress that only about five out of every hundred sufferers will develop serious disease with extensive disability. Another five patients in that same hundred may end up with some disability.

Out of any hundred sufferers from rheumatoid arthritis, about thirty can expect their disease either to disappear after a brief illness of several months duration; or else they will recover completely within a few years and be left with no resulting disablement. The remaining sixty or so patients can expect to have continuing trouble, with alternate flare-ups and remissions, for the rest of their lives.

What is the Conventional Medical Treatment?

Medical science has not yet discovered why the immune system, that usually so ably defends the body against infection, should suddenly turn aggressive and attack the joint tissues. Theories include an inherited predisposition and triggering factors such as viruses and various environmental conditions.

Conventional medicine, therefore, is still unable to come up with a cure for rheumatoid arthritis. It does however have a very great deal to offer in suppressing the worst symptoms of the disease, inhibiting its progress and preventing disability.

Drug therapy is a powerful weapon in the fight against rheumatoid arthritis. As it is the actual inflammation that causes the damage, anti-inflammatory drugs will help prevent further injury to the joints occurring. Painkillers may also be used, though to a very much more limited extent. Side-effects are an important factor in the use of drugs for this long-term illness; and the topic is discussed in Part Three of this book.

A careful regime, balancing adequate rest with exercise, is an essential ingredient of all programmes of treatment. The help of physiotherapists, occupational therapists and other specialists may be enlisted to safeguard the quality of life of the sufferer. The patient's GP is ideally placed to mobilise and co-ordinate these resources.

Surgery can also help by repairing snapped tendons, correcting deformities, removing inflamed synovial membranes and in replacing badly damaged joints.

Back Pain in General

The Spine

The human spine is a marvellously complex mechanism which often goes wrong. Conflicting reasons are advanced for this. Some maintain that the structure of the spine was evolved at a time when men walked on all fours, like four-legged animals, and that it is ill-suited to work in an upright position. Other experts reject that view entirely, believing that the spine is very well designed for its purpose and that it malfunctions only because of the bad habits imposed on it by modern living.

The spine serves several main functions. It gives shape to the body and supports its weight, together with any extra weight it may be carrying. It encases and protects the spinal cord, which is the main strand of nerves connecting the brain to all other parts of the body. The spine is so arranged as to allow the body to move in many directions, as well as keeping it stable during that movement. Not surprisingly, it is a complicated assembly of bones, joints, ligaments and other tissues.

An outline understanding of the arrangement of the bones and joints comprising the spine will be helpful before proceeding to read about some of the main rheumatic ailments that cause backache.

The Vertebrae

The spine consists of a large number of bones, *vertebrae* stacked one above the other. Each vertebra is connected to the one above and to the one below by three systems of joints.

The main part of a vertebra is a solid drum-shaped block of bone, facing the front of the body. This is called the *vertebral body* and carries the main weight.

Behind this and connected to it is a ring of bone with many protrusions, called the *neural arch*. Its shape is complex, which makes it difficult to show properly on a simple sketch. The neural arch faces the back of the body and its leading bony protrusion is what is felt by the fingers as they are run up and down the back.

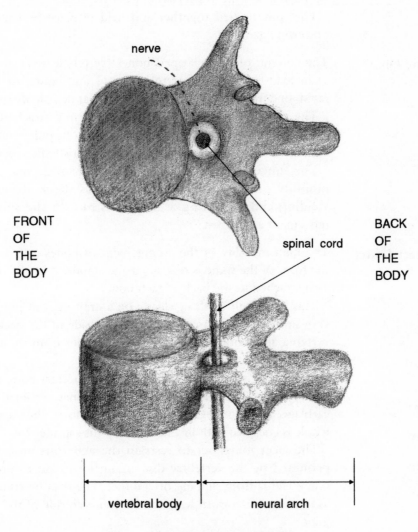

FRONT OF THE BODY

BACK OF THE BODY

nerve

spinal cord

vertebral body

neural arch

FIG. 2   TWO VIEWS OF A TYPICAL
VERTEBRA (simplified)

The spinal cord passes through a gap in the *neural arch* between it and the *main body* of each vertebra.

The spine is tied together and held in place by bands of powerful ligaments.

The Discs

The column of drum-shaped bones (vertebral bodies) is the main load-bearing part of the spine. These bones are separated, one from the other, by a series of flat flexible *discs*.

The top and bottom of each disc is firmly attached to a vertebra. The disc itself is composed of a soft, pulpy interior, contained within an outer lining of tough gristle-like tissue.

The function of the discs is both to provide maximum mobility to the vertebrae and to act as shock absorbers, yielding and distorting as weight is put on the spine in movement and at rest.

Facet Joints

The high mobility of the arrangement of bones and discs at the front of the spine is restrained and stabilised by the neural arch attached to the back of each bone.

This is difficult to show clearly on a drawing; but put at its very simplest, bony protrusions on each side of the back of a vertebra are connected to similar protrusions from the vertebrae above and below.

These *facet joints* as they are called, are normal body joints as shown in Figure 1. The ends of the bones are lined with cartilage, the joint spaces are filled with synovial fluid and the whole is enclosed with ligaments in a joint capsule.

The facet joints act to restrain the generous movement permitted by the vertebrae-disc arrangement and to prevent one vertebra from slipping off another. They can be visualised as two stabilising outriders, one pair on each side of the main joint.

A correctly aligned spine will carry the body's weight on the column formed by the front part of the vertebrae – the stack of solid bones and flexible discs. Bad distortion of spinal posture may tend to throw part of this weight backwards, on to the facet joints not intended for such purpose. Thinning or destruction of one or more discs may result in a local shortening of the spine and the jamming together of some of its

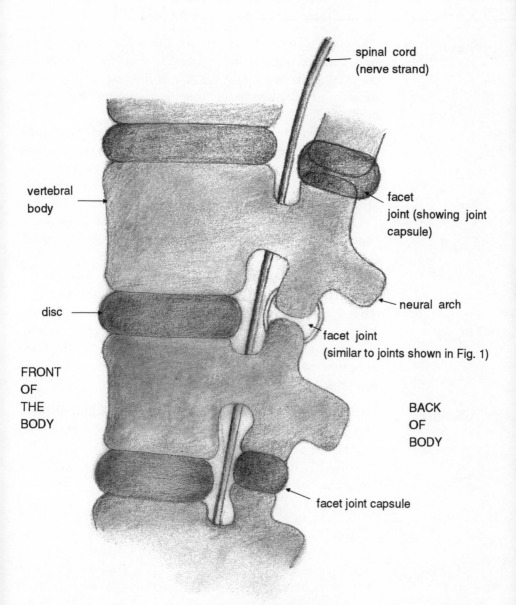

spinal cord
(nerve strand)

vertebral
body

facet
joint (showing joint
capsule)

disc

neural arch

facet joint
(similar to joints shown in Fig. 1)

FRONT
OF
THE
BODY

BACK
OF
BODY

facet joint capsule

Fig. 3   TYPICAL VERTEBRAE
(for clarity these are shown in much simplified outline and without their many
bony outcrops)

facet joints. Pain, stiffness and even permanent damage may result if these conditions are not corrected.

Nerves

The spinal cord passes through the gap between the front and back parts of the vertebrae. It is the main bundle of nerves connecting the brain with the rest of the body and is highly sensitive to any disturbance, reacting to pressure with severe pain.

As will be seen from the sketch, any gross distortion of the discs can put pressure on one side of the spinal cord. So too can swelling of the facet joint capsules press on the other side of the spinal cord. Thus disc trouble, described later, and arthritis in the facet joints can each cause agonising pain.

The facet joints in particular, being themselves richly supplied with nerves, are probably the commonest source of backache.

Other vulnerable nerves are those which branch off the spinal cord and proceed to the different parts of the body. They leave the spinal cord through short channels, formed where adjacent parts of the bony protrusions at the rear of successive vertebrae meet. Any slight distortion of the bone structure can thus interfere with these nerves, which pass right through the joints, and cause back pain.

Ailments

Osteoarthritis and rheumatoid arthritis, as described in previous chapters, can affect the joints of the spine as they do other joints in the body.

Some of the more common specific spinal arthritic complaints are described below.

Ankylosing Spondylitis

What is it?

This is an arthritic disease of the back. It is similar to rheumatoid arthritis – but it mainly affects younger men, attacking the lower back and tail-bone. The active phase ceases after a time; and though this may recur more than once, eventually the illness gradually subsides and disappears altogether.

Heredity

For reasons still unknown, nearly all sufferers from ankylosing spondylitis come from the 7% to 10% of the population with the inherited antigen HLA-B27 in the white cells of their blood. Of course, only a tiny minority of those carrying this antigen is ever affected. If a close relative has ankylosing spondylitis, one is more prone but by no means certain to contract the disease.

What Actually Happens?

Ankylosing spondylitis starts with inflammation of the joints of the spine, usually in the lower back. As in rheumatoid arthritis, the inflammation actually attacks and damages the components of the joint. It causes backache, with pain spreading to the buttocks and down the thighs.

Rib and breast-bone joints may also be affected, making it feel more difficult to breathe. Sometimes other joints such as the hip, shoulder, neck, ankle or knee become inflamed. Eyes can redden and heels become tender to the touch.

After a period of active illness, the inflammation gradually subsides and healing starts.

During the process, spurs of bone grow out of each side of the vertebrae, across the joint. They restrict movement further and tend to lock adjacent vertebrae together. If unchecked, this can lead to permanent stiffness and forward curvature of the spine.

Diagnosis and Treatment

The disease is difficult to diagnose at first and it may even take a year or two for its presence to be confirmed.

The initial period of inflammation is usually treated by a combination of rest, exercise and anti-inflammatory drugs.

It then becomes important to do one's utmost to maintain the mobility of the joints in order to prevent the stooping posture and permanently bent back so often seen in those who have had ankylosing spondylitis. Exercises – swimming is ideal – and physiotherapy, as well as close attention to correct posture, are the means employed for this.

Manipulation of inflamed neck and back joints can cause serious damage and must never be attempted.

More than 75% of those with ankylosing spondylitis will be able to stay at work and maintain a normal lifestyle.

Slipped Disc, Spondylosis and Non-specific Backache

General

These, like osteoarthritis, are not diseases but mechanical conditions caused by wear or damage to the joints of the spine.

They can be very troublesome and painful. Most sufferers recover completely in the end. But some do not; and have to treat their backs with special care for the rest of their lives.

The main parts of the vertebrae are separated from each other by flat flexible discs containing a soft pulpy substance within a tough outer casing of gristle. See the earlier chapter on Back Pain in General.

The function of the discs is to absorb the stresses, strains and shocks to which the back is constantly subjected. They also permit the mobility of the spine by allowing each vertebra to move freely against its two neighbours.

The processes of ageing often make the discs less able to play their part as intended. They become more vulnerable to damage in use, especially during the lifting of heavy objects.

Slipped Disc

When this happens, the outer casing of a disc tears, allowing part of the jelly-like substance inside to squeeze out. This forces the ligaments (binding the vertebrae together) to bulge inwards locally, sometimes pressing on one of the highly sensitive nerves from the spinal cord. Further movement is agonising.

This is the condition generally known as a *slipped disc*, though it would be better described as a torn (or prolapsed) disc.

Spondylosis This is another condition caused by degeneration of the discs. In spondylosis, the discs become thinner – as does the cartilage in ordinary osteoarthritis – and less flexible. The lower back or the neck may be affected by this complaint.

The spaces between the vertebrae narrow, causing stiffness. The vertebrae sometimes also grow bony spurs at their ends in an effort to compensate for the loss of disc effectiveness. These cause even more stiffness and may press on sensitive nerves.

Treatment for Slipped Disc and Spondylosis Treatment varies from patient to patient. A combination of rest and suitable exercise is usually all that is required, assisted by mild pain-killing drugs and other common sense remedies. Physiotherapy, steroid injections and even traction are sometimes suggested. The use of special corsets is best avoided. Surgical intervention may be necessary in a few cases.

Non-specific Backache There are other back and neck pains, which clear up on their own after sensible rest and care, for which no specific cause is ever found. These often occur as the result of a sudden awkward movement or unaccustomed exertion causing minor damage to the ligaments or joints of the spine. The majority of back pain falls into this category.

Strained muscles, or even emotional stress and worry, can also cause painful spasms which persist for days. Medical advice should be sought promptly if back pain does not subside and then cease altogether in reasonable time.

Other Less Common Forms of Arthritis

Psoriatic Arthritis

This is a special kind of arthritis which sometimes affects sufferers from psoriasis, a common non-infectious skin complaint which causes scaly patches. It tends to run in families.

The symptoms are not unlike those of rheumatoid arthritis; but they occur only in a few joints. The knees and back are the most vulnerable. Finger and toe nails often thicken, develop pits and change colour. Treatment is similar to that for the other forms of inflammatory arthritis. The psoriasis (of the skin) will of course have to be treated separately.

Reactive Arthritis (Reiter's Syndrome)

As its name suggests, this kind of arthritis occurs in reaction to an infection. Food poisoning, dysentery, rheumatic fever or some of the sexually transmitted illnesses can sometimes trigger reactive arthritis. This usually starts within a month or so of the infection first developing.

As in ankylosing spondylitis, it is those who carry the inherited HLA-B27 antigen who are most likely to contract this kind of arthritis. The reason for this is unknown.

Reiter's disease is the combination of urethritis (penile discharge), arthritis and conjunctivitis (painful eyes). It usually starts with pain and swelling in the knee or the ball of the foot, often followed by pain in the lower back. Tendons as well as joints may become inflamed; and this can result, for example, in badly swollen toes and tender heels. Further attacks of eye inflammation are also possible, as well as flaking of the skin in patches, rather like psoriasis.

The good news is that this type of arthritis is seldom severe and often affects only one or two joints. Also, for the large majority of patients, it clears itself up naturally during the course of several months. Only about ten per cent sustain significant joint damage or continuing arthritic attacks.

The first essential in any kind of treatment is to clear up the underlying infection with antibiotics. Thereafter, drugs are avoided in most cases, with the condition being left to cure itself. Mobility is preserved and permanent damage to the joints avoided by the same means used to treat other forms of arthritis.

Gout

Gout is predominantly an illness suffered by men. It rarely affects women, and then only after the menopause. A tendency to suffer from gout can be inherited. Gout is perhaps the most painful of all rheumatic diseases and the only one that can be entirely suppressed by drugs.

Gout is caused by too much uric acid in the blood forming itself into crystals which are then deposited in a joint. It is those crystals that cause the inflammation and pain.

Everyone has uric acid in his or her bloodstream and the body normally disposes of any excess without trouble. It is the breakdown of that system of natural elimination which causes the symptoms of gout.

Attacks of gout may be triggered by injuring a joint or by excessive drinking. Contrary to popular belief, gout is usually caused by a combination of an inherent tendency to the disease and simple bad luck. The joint of the big toe is the most likely to suffer; but the knee, the elbow and the wrist may also be vulnerable. A gouty joint swells suddenly, reddens and becomes excruciatingly tender. Crystals may also be deposited beneath the skin in what looks like a series of white pimples, mainly on the lobes of the ears and on the fingers.

Acute attacks may be relieved quickly by taking an anti-inflammatory drug such as Indomethacin.

Special diets are useful for long-term control; for it is sensible to avoid those foods that encourage the build up of uric acid. But the main treatment consists of regular doses of a drug – Allopurinol – to regulate uric acid levels in the blood. In serious cases this has to be taken permanently to prevent symptoms from returning; but such treatment can only start after the acute attack has abated.

The latest drugs used for the treatment of gout are safe but some may cause irritating side effects.

Though gout is not curable, its symptoms can be totally suppressed.

Various Forms of Rheumatism

Polymyalgia Rheumatica (P M R)

P M R , as this is often called, affects people over the age of fifty. It attacks the muscles – especially those in the shoulders, arms and thighs – making them painfully stiff and difficult to move, especially in the early mornings. Much of the pain experienced is due to the inflammation of the blood vessels supplying the muscles.

The illness is accompanied by a general feeling of tiredness and sometimes by a slight fever. There may also be inflammation of the scalp and temples, as well as interference with vision.

Quite distinct from other forms of rheumatism, P M R can be diagnosed by blood test.

The symptoms respond dramatically to treatment by steroids (cortisone-type drugs); and this is usually maintained until the disease finally fades away of its own accord. It almost always disappears completely within a year.

Systemic Lupus Erythematosis (S L E)

This is yet another of the diseases in which the body's own immune system goes berserk and actually attacks the tissues of the body.

Its commonest features are fever, arthritis, rheumatism, round skin patches, rashes and kidney problems. A blood test can help confirm the diagnosis.

S L E can also affect many organs and parts – heart, lungs, kidneys, arteries and nervous system.

Permanent damage to the joints is rarely caused by lupus. Drugs are used to suppress the inflammation and help sufferers maintain mobility during more severe spells. S L E can be a mild disease, with its sufferers experiencing long periods of good health between bouts.

Occupational Rheumatism

Joints, tendons and muscles can all be affected by the strain caused by the frequent repetition of some routine operation or, for example, by constant use of an unsuitable chair. Factory workers, typists and musicians are only some of the many who may suffer from this type of complaint.

The worst symptoms can always be relieved temporarily by the use of drugs. But a proper cure can only come from recognising precisely what is causing the trouble and then taking the necessary measures to avoid that particular movement or posture.

Other Soft-tissue Complaints

General

Pain felt in the muscles and tendons is often caused by mild strain or even by stress due to anxiety. It has been given a variety of names – such as fibrositis, tendinitis, etc.

Most such conditions clear up themselves after a period of rest. If they do not, and if they persist for more than a few weeks, medical advice should be sought.

Frozen Shoulder

A slight injury to the shoulder, or even unaccustomed exercise, may bring on this condition. When it happens, inflammation around the shoulder joint produces a lot of pain which greatly restricts mobility – hence the name *frozen shoulder.* The joint itself is not damaged; but damage can occur if full movement of the shoulder is not restored before long. Therefore medical advice and treatment is necessary.

Tennis Elbow and Golfer's Elbow

In this case, the pain is caused by a damaged tendon in the elbow. If the one on the outside of the joint is affected, the patient has *Tennis Elbow:* damage to the one on the inside is called *Golfer's Elbow.* The injection of a steroid is often very effective in cases that do not respond quickly to simple rest and support.

Bursitis

The bursa is a small sack of fluid, located close to a joint. Its purpose is to ease movement of the skin and tendons over a bony projection such as at a joint.

When a bursa is injured or inflamed, excess fluid collects and causes a painful swelling. This usually subsides within a very few weeks and has no lasting effect.

The bursa most commonly affected are at the knee cap – *Housemaid's Knee* – the elbows, the shoulders and the heels.

Osteoporosis

This is only indirectly related to rheumatic disease. For those with osteoporosis, the thinning of the bones that happens normally with advancing age is greatly accelerated. Women are protected by oestrogen from this effect until the menopause, after which the process can suddenly increase in pace.

One result is a far greater vulnerability to accidental fractures. Another is that bones in the spine can simply crush under the body's weight, causing permanent stiffness and stooping. That kind of distortion can sometimes exert pressure on the bladder and the bowels.

Hormone replacement therapy after the menopause has proved very effective in delaying the onset of osteoporosis; but this protection ceases after H R T is discontinued. Proper diet, with an adequate intake of calcium, and sensible exercise routines, are also recommended.

Part Three

Conventional Management

In General

The causes of arthritis are still unknown and no cure for it has yet been found. But modern medical science now has a great deal to offer in ways of managing the symptoms of rheumatic disease and maintaining an adequate quality of life.

The latest techniques and therapies recommended by the best medical practice are outlined below.

Some involve highly specialised treatment, such as the use of powerful drugs. But others, based on good sense and general health care, have much in common with some of the better alternative therapies described in Part Four of this book.

Medical Advice

The Family Doctor

For most people, the first point of contact with the medical profession is their own family doctor.

The typical sufferer from rheumatic disease needs a great deal of skilled and patient care over long periods. Family doctors will very often be able to provide such help. They may refer their patients to specialists (rheumatologists) and to therapists (both physio' and occupational), whilst themselves providing constant guidance and support.

However there will always be a few doctors who, for one reason or another, lack the time, knowledge or patience to be able to provide exactly what is most needed. Worried beyond measure, and faced with a doctor who appears unsympathetic and brusque, what is the unfortunate sufferer to do ?

The best way to get better care is for the patient to voice his or her concerns frankly to the doctor. If the response is inadequate, the doctor should be changed for another who is more interested and communicative – but it is acknowledged that this is not always so easily done in the National Health Service.

Fortunately there are several outside organisations that can partly help to fill the gap.

Arthritis Care

Arthritis Care, which provides practical advice and information on how to cope with arthritis, has branches all over the country. It publishes a magazine and runs its own welfare department.

Families too are catered for in its extensive support operation. It runs specially equipped holiday centres and self-catering units for its members, as well as a small residential home for those who are very disabled.

Most important of all, its members are encouraged to keep in touch and derive mutual support and benefit from each other.

Arthritis Care can be contacted at its head office at 5 Grosvenor Crescent, London SW1X 7ER. Its telephone number is 071 235 0902.

The Arthritis and Rheumatism Council

The Council funds an extensive research programme and sponsors work of great value in that connection. It has produced a series of very worthwhile booklets on aspects of different forms of arthritis, rheumatism and connected ailments. It also publishes a magazine.

The Council can be reached at St. Mary's Court, St. Mary's Gate, Chesterfield, Derbyshire S41 7TD. Its telephone number is 0246 558033.

Other Associations

The Back Pain Association, Grundy House, 31 Park Road, Teddington, Middlesex TW11 OAB (tel. 081 977 5474), has local support branches all over the country. It supports research and provides advice and information to sufferers.

The National Ankylosing Spondylitis Association and *The Disabled Living Foundation* perform a similar function in providing a forum for researchers and sufferers alike, as well as offering practical help.

Further details of The Disabled Living Foundation are given in the later chapter on Managing Arthritis. The National Ankylosing Spondylitis Foundation can be contacted at 6 Grosvenor Crescent, London SW1X 7ER (tel. 071 235 9585).

**Special
Arthritis
Clinics**

There are now many out-patient rheumatology clinics in this country able to provide a fuller range of treatment, therapy, help, counselling and support to sufferers from arthritis – on the comprehensive lines offered by some clinics in the United States. These are attached to main hospitals and patients are referred to them by their GP.

A charity called *Arthritis Action* has also done valuable pioneering work in supporting specialised arthritis clinics within the National Health Service. Centred on the Christchurch Hospital, the local arthritis clinics of East Dorset are now providing just that form of overall care considered so valuable by patients. Arthritis Action has embarked on an extensive educational programme, in the hope of spreading this particular combination of specialised therapies outside its own area. Progress may be slow – but it is happening.

**Specialist
Hospitals**

The Horder Centre for Arthritis of St. John's Road., Crowborough, East Sussex TN6 1XP (Tel. 0892 665577), provides short and long term programmes of care and rehabilitation on an in-patient and out-patient basis. It also has a specialist surgical unit for NHS patients and others.

Several other specialist hospitals exist to provide therapy and rehabilitation for sufferers from arthritis. Patients may be sent on to such hospitals by the rheumatologist (specialist consultant) to whom they were originally referred by their general practitioner. Courses of exercises and other therapies at these hospitals, including those done under water (hydrotherapy), of from one to three weeks' duration can produce excellent results.

Partnership

It is important to remember that the fight against arthritis cannot be undertaken alone. It is a serious long-term engagement, requiring the unremitting participation of the patient as well as specialist guidance from doctors and therapists.

States of Mind

In General
From no part of this book will a reader get the impression that arthritis is in any way trivial or is something that can effortlessly be overcome if sufferers follow a particular course of treatment.

On the contrary, arthritis can be a scourge. It is a serious matter for those involved, often bringing months if not years of pain and disability in its wake. For a tiny minority, it can involve permanent disablement.

It is not surprising therefore that the onset of arthritis can provoke extreme anxiety. Those who get an acute form of the illness when young often feel cut off from active life in the flower of their youth. And those who contract it later on are sometimes overcome by a gloomy vision of steady deterioration with advancing age.

If this book has a single message, it is that both the over-pessimistic and the over-optimistic views are exaggerated. Arthritis is very serious for some; but with modern medicine and therapy, most of its worst effects can be mitigated sufficiently to maintain a satisfactory lifestyle.

The sufferer from arthritis will have to work continuously to obtain such relief. And that can only be done in a state of mind free from unreasonable worry, panic and depression.

Pain
The fear of pain itself causes even more pain. And that vicious cycle can often lead to panic or even to depression.

Depression
Depression is a state that is not always recognised as an illness by those affected; and such recognition is the first step to a cure. If someone awakens from sleep at four o'clock every morning in sheer panic and utter misery – if he or she loses interest in life, becomes permanently tired, listless and irritable – that person is probably suffering from depression.

Depression must be conquered as a first step to the positive thinking needed for effective therapy. It must be recognised for what it is; and every effort must be made to emerge from beneath its cloud. Such advice is easily given – but very much harder to carry out.

Fears and problems should be talked over freely with doctors or anyone prepared to listen. Most people have suffered from depression at some time in their lives and will be sympathetic. The more such worries can be discussed with others the better.

Few things in life can really be as bad as they may seem at four o'clock in the morning. Eventually the cloud will lift and more reasonable thoughts prevail over panic and despair. In extreme cases, sufferers should not hesitate to appeal for help to the Samaritans or to another emergency lifeline which exists for that purpose.

Daily life must be picked up again. As much activity as possible should be planned, especially that involving other people. It helps always to have things to do and to occupy the mind, as well as some event to which one can look forward.

Depression really can be eliminated by determined effort and the help of others. The major task of living with arthritis can then be tackled in earnest.

Drugs

The use of tranquillisers and sleeping pills should first be cut down and then eliminated altogether as soon as practicable. They often cause depression. So too does heavy drinking.

Some of the newer anti-depressant drugs tend to be less addictive and have fewer side-effects than those previously in use. Clinical trials have shown then to be effective in many cases.

Over-anxiety

Over-anxiety, as opposed to depression, also feeds on itself and inhibits effective therapy. A certain amount of worry is natural. Too much is harmful.

A good way of banishing unreasonable anxiety is to acquire knowledge of the condition and to attempt fuller under-standing of what is involved. This can be done in discussion with doctors, therapists and fellow sufferers, as well as by asking questions and reading about it. The illness will then assume realistic proportions in the mind, allowing positive attitudes to overcome irrational fears.

Diet

General Advice

Many claims are made by practitioners of alternative therapies for the value of certain diets in treating and even curing rheumatic disease (see Part Four of this book). A powerful case is also made out by those who believe in a close connection between allergy and arthritis (see Part Five). Nevertheless, conventional medical opinion remains deeply sceptical except in cases of gout.

Some doctors acknowledge that, for a very few people, a diet free from dairy products may assist. Again, short-term relief from the inflammation associated with rheumatoid arthritis can be obtained by fasting – though this wears off as soon as normal eating is resumed.

A general warning must be given here against any diet that does not provide a well-balanced range of foods and sufficient calories to maintain health. An arthritis sufferer has quite enough to cope with already without adding undernourishment to the many other problems.

There are two aspects of dieting on which all are agreed. The first is that a well-balanced diet will promote general health and must be beneficial. The second is that excessive body weight should be avoided as this puts extra stress on critical joints.

Gout

As described in Part Two of this book, the symptoms of gout are caused by uric acid in the blood being deposited as crystals in certain joints.

It makes sense therefore to reduce dependence on drugs to control uric acid levels by avoiding foods known to be rich in substances contributing to this effect.

Alcohol – beer and heavy red wines in particular, liver and bacon, roes including caviar, and sardines and cod are some of the commoner foods to be avoided where possible.

Being Overweight

It is estimated that, when walking, the knee and hip joints carry up to five times the body weight. One extra pound in weight will therefore add the equivalent of about five pounds in stress to the hips and knees.

41

Reducing weight to recommended levels makes a lot of sense for sufferers from arthritis. It will ease pressure on the joints, improve mobility, lessen pain and also benefit the sufferer's general health.

Much has been written elsewhere on the problem of losing weight. All that is added here is that this should be done slowly, methodically and with care. A family doctor will often be able to recommend a suitable diet or refer the patient to a nutritionist for more specialist guidance.

Special crash diets are not recommended; and advice should always be taken to ensure that no elements necessary for a balanced diet are cut out in the process.

Joining an association such as Weight Watchers, where problems, successes and failures may be shared with others, is recommended as one possible solution for those who might respond to this kind of support.

Low-fat Diets

Such diets substitute polyunsaturated vegetable and fish oils for the saturated fat contained in animal products such as red meat, butter and milk.

This type of diet is, of course, recommended by doctors as a means of reducing heart disease. But in so far as arthritis is concerned, the advice given by the Arthritis and Rheumatism Council for Research is only that *it may help a little in cases of arthritis.*

Deficiencies

Medical opinion is that vitamin and mineral deficiencies which can affect arthritis are rare in those who maintain a balanced diet. Reliance on dietary supplements is not, in general, encouraged.

High doses of steroids sometimes used to treat rheumatoid arthritis can induce calcium deficiency. This must be remedied promptly before the bones thin and lose weight.

The use of certain other drugs may very occasionally require a low-salt diet. In that case, sodium products – common salt, sodium bicarbonate, sodium benzoate, monosodium glutamate – should be avoided and all food content labels checked for their presence.

Food Allergy Conventional medical opinion denies that allergy can cause arthritis, though some rheumatologists acknowledge that *a very few patients* show improvement when certain foods are cut out of their diet. The reader is referred to Part Five of this book for further information and for sharply conflicting views.

Drug Therapy

In General Drugs are a powerful weapon in the struggle to minimise the effects of arthritis – but they must be used with care.

The prolonged use of drugs is controversial, even within the medical profession. Of course they can save life and greatly relieve the pain and suffering associated with rheumatic disease. On the other hand, nearly all drugs are to a greater or lesser extent toxic to the patient; and some reactions to their use can be life-threatening.

Side-effects Apart from the beneficial effect of a particular drug on the symptoms for which it has been prescribed, it may also affect other parts of the body. The results of this, when irritating or harmful, are called side-effects.

Eventually every drug will produce some side effects, tolerable or otherwise, when the patient has had enough of it. The severity of the adverse reaction will be increased by large doses and also if the drug is taken for a long time.

It is important to remember that not everyone reacts in the same way to any drug. It is possible that when one produces an unpleasant reaction, another in the same group may not. Reaction to drugs must be monitored and changes made at once if necessary.

A careful balance must be kept when considering the use of drugs and their side-effects. Many people are totally dependent on drugs to maintain their mobility. For them, the side-effects, however unpleasant, are a price that it is very well worth paying.

Pain-killers (analgesics)

These are most often used in the treatment of osteoarthritis, and soft-tissue rheumatic complaints. They are best reserved for short-term problems and for peaks of acute pain.

When used for rheumatoid arthritis, care must be taken not to damage swollen joints by too much movement. Pain is the usual warning signal that damage is being caused – but this will have been masked by the effect of a drug.

The simplest pain-killing remedy in everyday use consists of one or two tablets of paracetamol – increasingly preferred to aspirin as it does not irritate the stomach as much. Even paracetamol can cause great harm in overdose; and in no circumstances should more than eight tablets be taken in any one day.

Various stronger preparations, such as Copraxamol, are available on prescription to treat severe pain. These can cause constipation and tiredness but few present real problems in occasional use.

The most powerful pain-killing drugs of all, such as morphine and pethidine, are reserved for emergencies and have little place in arthritic treatment.

Anti-inflammatory Drugs

These are used mostly to reduce the damaging inflammation caused in rheumatoid arthritis and related complaints.

Aspirin used to be the most popular; but it has to be taken in such large quantities (12 to 14 tablets a day) that its side-effects – particularly on the stomach – can cause trouble.

Drug companies have therefore produced a large number of substitutes to reduce inflammation with fewer disadvantages.

These are known as non-steroidal anti-inflammatory drugs (NSAIDs). As their commonest side-effect is stomach irritation, they are always taken after meals. Suppositories, such as Voltarol, are also available; and these have fewer side-effects.

NSAIDs can also cause rashes, irritation, dizziness and ringing in the ears of some patients. Their prolonged use is a matter of trial and error and is becoming increasingly controversial.

Second-line Drugs

Penicillamine, Sulphasalazine, Hydroxychloroquine and gold salts are powerful drugs used to reduce inflammation in rheumatoid arthritis and (hopefully) to modify the course of the disease.

They all take some time to take effect and a course lasting for six months is usually the minimum. The resulting benefit should persist for at least a year after the end of the treatment, and possibly for up to three or four years after that.

The downside is that these drugs are very toxic and experience has shown that at least half of all patients will discontinue their use within twelve months because of adverse effects. The drugs can damage the kidneys and the bone marrow though this is reversed after the cessation of treatment, if damage has not progressed too far. Their use is therefore very carefully monitored by blood testing.

Other side-effects can include skin rashes. Damage to blood cells may inhibit blood clotting and also make the body vulnerable to infection. Some people may also get mouth ulcers and feel sick.

Steroids (cortisone-type drugs)

These powerful drugs, which affect the body's immune system, can be very helpful and even life-saving on occasion. They can also be dangerous. They are therefore only given for specific indications and are rarely used for more general conditions such as rheumatoid arthritis.

Steroids, such as Prednisolone, are usually taken by mouth for long periods.

Steroids are used in the treatment of P M R. The doses must continue for about three years if profound wastage of muscles is to be avoided. If the eyesight is threatened, the dosage is increased until blood tests show that the condition is under control. In these cases, steroids will save a person's sight.

Severe cases of S L E , in which the lungs or the heart are involved, also respond well to steroid treatment.

Injections of a steroid into a swollen and painful joint can provide instant relief for conditions like Tennis Elbow. By temporarily removing pain and inflammation, the joint is enabled to heal itself naturally with the help of suitable exercise. This is not repeated more than once or twice in any one joint for fear of doing damage.

The side-effects of taking steroids can be serious. They increase with the size of the doses and the length of time during which they are administered. Too much steroid can cause ulcers and skin rashes, puffiness and increased hairiness of the face, bruising of the skin, high blood pressure and diabetes.

Steroids inhibit the functioning of the adrenal gland, which produces its own natural steroids for the body. The gland slowly shrinks with their use, thus causing increasing dependency on the drug. Long terms of treatment may therefore be interrupted periodically to allow the gland to recover. But as taking the drug must never be abruptly terminated, users are encouraged to carry warning cards on their persons wherever they go.

Further Reading

Those interested in reading further are directed to two sources, each representing a different view of the use of drugs.

Drugs and Arthritis. Information Sheet published by the Arthritis and Rheumatism Council, Copeman House, St. Mary's Court, St. Mary's Gate, Chesterfield, Derbyshire S41 7TD. Telephone 0256 558033

Rheumatoid Arthritis. The Treatment Controversy. Edited by Goddard and Butler and published by Macmillan.

Rest and Exercise, Heat and Hydrotherapy

In General

Rest and exercise, in balanced amounts, are both essential in the treatment of arthritis. A patient will need far more rest than an average healthy person – and this must never be denied.

On the other hand, joints that are not moved regularly may deform or seize up permanently. Neglected muscles will waste away. And a minimum amount of exercise is needed to maintain general body fitness beneficial to all.

A certain amount of exercise therefore is vital to prevent the disability that, in past years, so often resulted from arthritis. However, exercise can be painful and even harmful if misused.

Heat and water therapy can be used to assist in moving stiff and painful joints.

Rest

One or two weeks of rest in bed is often indicated during acute phases of rheumatoid arthritis. Then, arms and legs may also be forcibly rested by the use of splints.

Other sufferers from rheumatic disease would be wise always to take a number of short rest periods during the course of each day. They must learn to accept that adequate rest is necessary for their condition and that such patterns of relaxation will help prevent them from becoming over-tired.

Sleep

A good sleep every night helps greatly in keeping excessive fatigue at bay and fostering a positive mental state. Again, this must be planned carefully – for sound sleep can be elusive.

Though an occasional sleeping pill may be useful as a *crutch*, it should never be taken regularly. In the medium and long term, sleeping pills will do more harm than good.

The patient would do better to rely instead on achieving the right physical and mental conditions to induce sleep. Though these may have to be worked at, nothing worthwhile comes without effort.

It is important to establish a regular sleeping pattern, with set hours, and to try to keep to this as far as possible.

A firm mattress is essential. Its effect can be enhanced at low cost by the use of a sheet of 12 mm thick chipboard under the mattress. The pillow should be flat. Warm bedclothes and the use of an electric blanket can help.

Tea, coffee and too much alcohol should be avoided for some hours before bedtime. A warm bath is soothing. If painkillers or anti-inflammatory drugs are prescribed, these should be taken last thing at night with a warm, bland drink.

Again, the mind should not be over-stimulated before sleep; and the latter part of every evening is best spent free from too much excitement. Stress and anxiety must be left behind for the night. Reading or music will often encourage drowsiness.

Worry about not sleeping is often itself a cause of insomnia. It should be remembered that most people need far less sleep as they grow older.

Relaxation Relaxation techniques can be useful, both in inducing sleep at night and in making the most of rest periods during the day. Even if complete mastery takes a little time, the techniques are simple and easily learned.

Many books are available describing different relaxation methods in detail. The principles, however, are simple.

First, a suitable environment must be found – warm and quiet with no distractions, and with a comfortable armchair, sofa or bed. Only then can the process of relaxation start. Also, this should not be attempted too soon after eating.

One popular method is very similar to that used in meditation. Sitting comfortably, first the eyes are closed. All the muscles of the body are then relaxed – quite consciously, progressing from limb to limb and finally ending with the neck and face. It sometimes helps to tense each group of muscles before relaxing them.

Deep breathing then starts, slowly and regularly. Breath is drawn in through the nose, down into the diaphragm. The breath is held for about five seconds and then expelled equally slowly though parted lips. Full attention should be given to the mechanics of breathing; and the hands, placed on the abdomen, will constantly monitor its steady rise and fall as each breath is taken and then expelled.

The mind must be cleared of all distracting thoughts, both at the beginning and when they occur later on. It should be concentrated on a single sound – say, a long drawn out *Ou..ou..mm* – repeated silently during each breathing-out operation.

The process is continued for about twenty minutes; and the subject remains at rest with eyes closed for another few minutes after that.

Other methods may be tried if this particular one does not work after practising for a week or two.

However, it must be recognised that relaxation is not always easy to achieve, especially if self-taught without expert guidance. Ideally a teacher should be found to impart the necessary technique, either individually or in classes run periodically in most cities for that purpose.

Joint Mobility Exercises

Joints will seize up and become permanently deformed or fixed in position if not used regularly. Suitable exercise is therefore a most important component of all methods of treating arthritis and lessening its effects.

Those with arthritis should at once start exercising their joints through their full ranges of movement. This should be done several times a day. The aim is to move a joint as far as it will go without causing much pain; and then to try coaxing it just a little further.

All kinds of methods may be used to assist. For example, heat can be applied first; or the exercises can be done in water. See later sections of this book on heat, cold and hydro therapies.

Care must be taken not to damage the swollen *hot* joints encountered during acute phases of rheumatoid arthritis. But some joint movement is equally necessary here, despite the difficulty – and even for joints being *rested* in splints.

Cold packs are often useful before attempting to move *hot* joints – a packet of frozen peas, for example, can be most effective.

The type and degree of exercise to be undertaken by some of those with arthritis can be a problem; for movement, essential though it is, causes pain and can even do harm unless undertaken under skilled direction.

Several books describe excellent exercise programmes for different conditions. One of the best is *The Arthritis Helpbook* by Kate Lorig and James F. Fries. This is published in this country by the Souvenir Press and is based on regimes developed at the Stanford Arthritis Center in California.

However all exercise programmes must be set up and supervised by a physiotherapist with special knowledge of the particular condition. Books should be used only for further information and reference.

Muscle Strengthening Muscles and tendons will weaken and waste away if not used constantly, thus subjecting the joints to even more pressure and damage.

Similar exercises exist to maintain and strengthen muscles as to maintain joint mobility. As advised in the above paragraph, a physiotherapist should prescribe a suitable programme. The book recommended above is also very useful.

Keeping Fit This too is important to maintain general health and alertness. Any programme should contain a due proportion of exercises designed to promote overall fitness.

Postural Education & Manipulation Special courses of lessons and exercises are beneficial to those with back complaints. They are designed to correct and prevent spinal deformity.

Manipulation of damaged or displaced joints, especially of the spine, can bring much relief if carried out carefully after proper medical diagnosis of the condition. Unskilled, blind manipulation should never be attempted.

Here again, a skilled physiotherapist should be consulted. The alternative therapies that deal with posture, described in Part Four of this book, can be regarded as *complementary* rather than *alternative* in so far as posture is concerned.

Heat Therapy This takes many forms. It is soothing and helpful for all cases of rheumatism and arthritis, other than during acute stages of rheumatoid arthritis when the joints are hot and inflamed. Heat therapy can be used simply to relieve pain and also before exercise.

Heat can be applied directly to a troubled joint by means of dry packs, moist packs or a radiant lamp.

Short wave diathermy and microwave diathermy both cause waves of energy to penetrate the tissues where they are converted into heat.

Ultrasonic rays effect the same kind of heating but also have some mechanical effect within the tissues or joints. They are not useful in cases of chronic arthritis.

Cold Therapy

The inflamed, hot joints encountered during acute phases of rheumatoid arthritis can be eased by the application of ice packs or similar means.

Again, this can assist the minimum exercise necessary even for joints that have been temporarily immobilised for the purpose of rest.

Hydrotherapy

Bathing in, and drinking, certain spring waters has been used as a means of therapy in famous spas since ancient times. This treatment, supplemented by mud baths, etc., is still available today in British and continental spas. It is regarded as an addition to conventional medicine for those who appreciate such treatment and think they derive benefit from it.

Of more direct use to sufferers from arthritis are the courses of exercises that are carried out under water at such places and elsewhere. This method is particularly helpful because as the water supports much of the weight of the body, stress in the joints is greatly reduced, permitting a wider range of movement with less pain.

Joint Protection

In General

An important part of the process of overcoming arthritis is to learn to adapt to living with its symptoms. Those with stiff and painful joints would be foolish indeed to try to ignore them. Far better to understand the limitations imposed by the condition and develop sensible patterns of daily life to suit.

The aim should be to avoid putting too much stress on vulnerable joints by allowing other parts of the body to do more of the work. Movements should be consciously planned in such a way as to conserve energy by avoiding wasteful effort.

Expert Advice

Books are available in popular bookshops which give detailed advice on determining which particular movements cause most pain and how best to modify them.

Methods of lifting, carrying, sitting and walking are described, together with a variety of alternative ways of performing simple tasks at work, in the home or in the garden to cause the least stress and pain. One of the best of these is *The Arthritis Helpbook* by Kate Lorig and James Fries, published by Souvenir Press.

Very often an occupational therapist will be able to give valuable advice.

The Disabled Living Foundation, with branches all over the country, has trained staff to provide guidance on the many different appliances available to help. Its head office is at 380 Harrow Road, London W9 2HU. Telephone: 071 289 6111.

Arthritis Care can also help. Its particulars are included in the last chapter.

Main Guidelines

These will depend to a large extent on which joints are affected. Though techniques are mostly a matter of common-sense, it is sometimes surprising how much even the simplest device can assist.

For example, the use of a walking stick can greatly relieve the load on a leg or foot joint. Those with shoulder, neck or back trouble should avoid carrying heavy objects and should use a trolley instead – such as a shopping trolley on wheels. Sufferers from backache should not lift heavy objects; and when lifting is done, it should be by bending the knees instead of the back.

Cushioned shoes, such as those worn by joggers, greatly reduce the jolting effect of normal walking on hip, knee, ankle and foot joints. They should be worn whenever possible. Another useful principle is to use the strongest or largest joint available. If the fingers are weak, the palm of the hand or the whole arm should be used instead. Both arms should be employed where possible, instead of just one arm. When rising from a sitting position, both feet should press firmly on the floor and both arms be used for leverage.

Storage in the kitchen and elsewhere should be adapted for ease of access without necessitating awkward or difficult movements. Bathrooms can be adapted with grab rails to ease getting in and out of the bath, or up from the toilet seat. Taking a shower can be an easier alternative to taking a bath.

Long handles can be fitted to household and garden tools and appliances. Simple gadgets can be fitted to facilitate the turning of taps. In the car, specially wide rear mirrors to reduce having to turn the neck, power-assisted brakes and steering can make a lot of difference.

Specially adapted clothing, with velcro fasteners instead of zips, etc., can be obtained by mail order. See the catalogues issued by J.D. Williams and Co. Ltd., 53 Dale Street, Manchester M60 1UH.

The list of such simple hints may seem endless. But skilled guidance from experts and from books really will help.

The Feet

The feet, often a source of pain and discomfort to those with arthritis, deserve careful attention. One rheumatologist reported recently that half of a large sample of patients with arthritis was found to be in need of chiropody.

Shoes

A great deal can be done with shoes to minimise pain and inconvenience – even simple inserts and insoles can bring relief. Of course, for women in particular, a change to a different type of shoe – for much, if not all the time – can bring dramatic relief in walking. Jogging shoes are the best. Specialist shops, such as Scholls, are able to give good practical advice.

For more pronounced deformity, made-to-measure shoes of quite acceptable appearance are now available, even on the National Health Service.

Sex and Parenthood

Anxiety

Lessening of the sexual urge because of worry about arthritis, as well as joint pain experienced during intercourse, are in themselves sources of anxiety to sufferers.

This type of stress, like many others, is lessened by fuller understanding of what is involved and by expert guidance.

There is no reason at all why those with arthritis should not enjoy an active sex life well into old age – if that is what they want. Indeed, arthritis should interfere as little as possible with normal life, of which sex can be an important part.

Sexual activity is certainly not harmful to sufferers from rheumatic disease. In fact it stimulates the body to produce adrenalin and other substances which help to relieve pain. So, from that point of view, the more sex the better!

Intercourse

People with damaged or inflamed joints – hip joints in particular – can experience much discomfort when attempting sexual intercourse in the *missionary* position (the man on top of the woman). There are, of course, several other positions that will be found easier and less painful.

Alternatives should be explored. Those in which the woman lowers herself on to the man, or those in which the partners lie side by side, one behind the other, are the most promising avenues for experiment.

Advice

For couples who have difficulty in discussing intimate matters with others, or even between themselves, skilled help really is needed. There is no shame, nor should there be undue embarrassment, in seeking help from doctors, therapists or medical social workers. Sexual activity is important for most people; and every effort should be made to maintain its quality.

The *Association of Sexual and Marital Therapy*, at P.O. Box 62, Sheffield S10 3TS, maintains a list of trained therapists able to advise on such problems.

Another organisation, formed to stimulate awareness of the sexual needs of disabled people and publicise measures which may be taken to alleviate their problems, is *The Association to Aid the Sexual and Personal Relationship of People with a Disability.* Its address is 286 Camden Road, London N7 OBJ.

Serious books on sexual techniques are readily available in the shops.

The Arthritis and Rheumatism Council also publishes a useful booklet on this subject with the primary aim of encouraging greater frankness and better communication in what for some is still a delicate subject. It is called *Arthritis: Sexual Aspects and Parenthood,* and may be obtained from the Council at St. Mary's Court, St. Mary's Gate, Chesterfield, Derbyshire S14 7TD (Tel. 0246 558033).

Surgery

As described in the later section on Surgery, a hip replacement operation will usually be able to restore the ability to have intercourse within a very few months.

Family Planning

The use of a coil (I.U.D.) should cause no problem for people with arthritis.

Nor should the *pill,* unless this interferes with an anti-arthritis drug being taken at the same time and blood pressure is raised. The doctor should always be consulted before this method of family planning is adopted.

Skilled advice from a Family Planning Clinic or doctor should be sought if arthritic joints make a cap or sheath difficult to use, when alternative methods may be suggested.

Heredity

Arthritis is not inherited directly, but those who carry a particular antigen in their white blood cells certainly are far more prone to some forms of the illness than the general population.

There is no compelling reason therefore to hesitate about having children on this account. It may however be reassuring to seek specialist advice in extreme cases.

Childbirth

A mother with badly deformed joints may require a different method of delivery as well as more care after the birth. Otherwise, childbirth should be normal.

Care of Children

An arthritic mother will always need more rest than a normally healthy woman. She should aim never to get too exhausted.

Bringing up children is strenuous as well as rewarding. The amount of help and support available from the husband and others is the main consideration in deciding when to have children and on the size of family.

Once the baby arrives, an occupational therapist will be able to advise on available means of looking after the infant without too much stooping and with the least strain.

All the same, arrangements must be made to enable the mother to get the rest she needs – including periods in bed if indicated. That is essential.

The Weather

Yes, there can be no doubt that the weather does affect those with rheumatic disease. Aches and pains are aggravated by cold, by humidity and by rapid changes in barometric pressure. The reasons for this may not be understood; but the effects are real enough. The sensitivity of arthritis sufferers to approaching thunderstorms is referred to again in Part Five of this book, where a possible explanation is offered.

A warm, dry environment is the best for arthritis sufferers. Those enjoying such conditions will generally experience less pain than others, with a similar complaint, living and working in cold or damp conditions. Humidity, even if combined with heat, will also tend to worsen the symptoms.

However, a pamphlet, issued in 1992 by the Arthritis and Rheumatism Council (address as given above), wisely warns sufferers against cutting themselves off from family and friends by going to live in a better climate abroad.

It draws attention to the fact that mental stress can have a similar effect on joints as that caused by cold and dampness. It concludes that it is probably better to live surrounded by family and friends in a warm, dry house in England than to flee to comparative isolation in sunny Spain. A combination of both is, of course, the ideal for those fortunate enough to be able to afford it.

Surgery

Though minor surgery, such as the repair of tendons, is often attempted, major surgery is not usually resorted to until other means have failed and disability is becoming a major problem.

Sometimes, paradoxically, joints can be improved by stiffening them. This kind of operation is known as arthrodesis. It relieves the pain at the cost of limiting full movement of a joint; and can be a preferable alternative to replacing the joint itself.

An operation called synovectomy, which may bring relief for several years, involves the complete removal of a chronically inflamed joint lining. This is only attempted when the joint itself has not been damaged. However, recovery from such operations is slow.

Badly deformed joints can sometimes be corrected by osteotomy. This involves cutting the bone without entering the joint itself. This is not a major surgical operation and its benefit can be long lasting.

The simplest form of joint replacement (excision arthroplasty) consists of removing the ends of the bones at a joint. It is often carried out on the ball of the foot and also at the wrist. Nature eventually replaces the missing bone ends with fibrous tissue and the results are usually worthwhile.

Joint Replacement

Complete replacement of a joint (arthroplasty) by a metal and plastic joint (prosthesis) is a major operation, only undertaken when the surgeon is convinced that it is justified.

Remarkable results are now obtained in replacing hip joints and similar operations on the knees have dramatically improved in recent years. The replacement of shoulder, elbow, knuckle and ankle joints has not yet been advanced to anything like the same degree.

As the life of such artificial joints in use has not yet been established beyond doubt, it is usual to delay such drastic surgery until the patient is over fifty-five years old.

As stated above, the success rate for hip operations is now very high indeed. But there is still, for some unknown reason, a risk of infection developing – which is perhaps the only cloud on the horizon. Patients with chronic infections in other parts of the body are therefore discouraged from undergoing this operation.

Further Reading

More useful information on this subject can be found in a booklet called *Arthritis and Joint Replacement* by Professor Verna Wright. This may be obtained direct from The Bookshop, British Medical Association, BMA House, Tavistock Square, London WC1 9JP. Tel. 071 387 4499.

Part Four

The Alternative Therapies

Underlying Ideas

The Difference

Most alternative therapies are based on an approach to health and sickness that differs sharply from that of conventional medicine – or at least of its more conservative wing. Some understanding of this fundamental difference should be gained before proceeding to details of those particular therapies claimed to be of benefit to sufferers from rheumatic disease.

Of course, the many so-called systems of alternative medicine themselves vary widely. Some, such as traditional Chinese medicine, are ancient indeed. Others, founded very much more recently, employ the tools of modern science to monitor vital bodily functions. Again, some forbid the use of drugs altogether, while others depend heavily on complex substances contained in herbs and natural extracts.

Health and Disease

However different the language of each discipline may be – whether the terms it uses are those of bodily meridians, yin and yang, or X-rays and blood pressure – a single thread of ideas is common to most of them.

It is the whole person, body and mind, that is the primary focus of diagnosis and treatment – and not just the particular ailment from which the person happens to be suffering. A human being is not seen as a machine, with one or two parts defective and in need of repair or replacement, but rather as a complex integrated whole.

In fact, the symptoms of disease are regarded as signs of a far deeper disturbance of the body's flow of vital energy and power of self-healing. Though bacteria, viruses and other external factors may also be significant, the causes of disease are far from simple. Many elements in a person's heredity and way of living play their part. These include smoking, faulty diet, bad posture and lack of correct exercise, acute emotional stress and many other abuses of body and mind.

Healing

It follows therefore that restoration to true health may also be more complex than the simple cures aimed for by conventional doctors.

Most systems of alternative medicine aim first to rid the patient of accumulated toxins, rebuild the natural balance and then replenish his or her reservoir of self-healing power. It is claimed that natural healing can proceed with best effect only after that has been accomplished.

This basic concept can be expressed in many different ways, depending on which language is used by the chosen system – but in practice, they all amount to very much the same kind of process. Correction of flows of vital energy, physical posture, muscular tension, nutritional balance and emotional stability are just some of the terms employed.

Some therapies also intervene directly in the healing process, tackling symptoms of disease by physical manipulation, acupuncture, herbs, homeopathic remedies and other means.

A combination of a basic purification and self-healing system with several of the directly interventionist therapies is usually of most help in cases of rheumatic disease.

Body and Mind

Mind and body are considered inseparable in the healing process.

Reasonable people acknowledge that, if the circumstances are right, the body will cure itself of most maladies. A cut finger, a feverish infection, a deep surgical incision, a joint mildly damaged by osteoarthritis, for example, will often mend without outside interference. Also, living cells in all parts of the human body are in a constant state of renewal, driven by some self-regulating mechanism.

It is increasingly accepted that people are especially vulnerable to disease when in a state of acute anxiety or depression. Emotional shocks, like the death of a loved one or an ill-planned retirement, can exact a heavy toll.

But until a few years ago it was considered eccentric in some orthodox medical circles to believe that the conscious mind can influence health directly, or indeed affect automatic functions such as pulse, temperature and blood pressure. Now that it appears to have been demonstrated beyond reasonable doubt that the mind can, if suitably mobilised, control some of these processes, the boundaries of what may be possible have moved.

Practitioners of biofeedback techniques have shown that the rate of breathing and heartbeat, the temperature and blood pressure, really can be altered and maintained in the new state for long periods by the use of the mind alone. Why, it is asked, cannot the body's power of self-healing also be stimulated in similar manner?

Placebo

The placebo effect – in which a patient recovers rapidly after receiving doses of what he or she believes to be a powerful drug but in fact is no more than coloured water – is an illustration of the power of mind over body. So too, as every parent who has *kissed better* a hurt child knows, does the caressing or the *laying-on* of hands, by someone in a position of trust and authority, serve to relieve pain.

External Healing Powers

As old as human history itself is the special gift of healing claimed by a few favoured individuals. The healer seeks to transfer part of his own healing power to augment the depleted resources of a sufferer, usually through physical contact by the laying-on of hands.

Another type of charismatic healer, very often religiously inspired, will attempt to harness some power outside himself for the same purpose. This can be done by a variety of means including prayer, sometimes assisted by physical contact.

There can be little doubt that, for whatever reason, such methods do sometimes work.

The Patient

It will be seen that, in most alternative therapies, the patient is not merely a passive recipient of treatment, waiting for some wonder drug to bring about a cure. Rather, he or she becomes a major participant in the twin tasks of trying to understand the causes of the disease and in undertaking a programme of self-healing – all initiated and guided by the therapist.

A similar attitude is also finding its way into conventional medicine – and especially for diseases like arthritis for which no cure can be offered. Indeed some of the latest so-called conventional methods for managing arthritis, described in Part Three of this book, owe a great deal to the very same kind of basic thinking.

Therapists, Diagnosis and Treatment

The Alternative Practitioner

Responsible therapists recognise the limitations of their own particular discipline and in some ways regard their efforts as complementary to conventional medicine.

They accept that they perform best with chronic ailments, like rheumatic disease, for which doctors can do little; and will refer acute disorders and injuries with which they cannot cope – particularly in children and the elderly – to an appropriate physician or surgeon.

An alternative therapist who is also medically trained will be in a particularly good position to recognise at once which conditions his therapy cannot treat.

It has been reliably estimated that the average alternative therapist spends between six and eight times the length of time on each patient as does the ordinary family doctor. As very little alternative medicine is available on the National Health Service, its use is expensive.

It is important to avoid quacks – not just because of the cost, but also because of the time lost and the inevitable disappointment involved. It may also be unsafe to undergo treatment at the hands of someone unskilled in his own discipline and uncertain of the boundaries of his own knowledge.

If personal recommendations from satisfied patients are not offered, expert guidance should be sought. Some qualifications may sound impressive but mean very little. Lists of reliable organisations to be consulted are included below, after the section on each therapy.

Diagnosis

A first session with an alternative practitioner will differ appreciably from that with most conventional doctors. The time taken, the scope of questions asked and the methods used for diagnosis may well seem bizarre to someone unfamiliar with alternative medicine.

The therapist, seeking to assess the condition of the patient, body and mind, and not just the symptoms of the illness, will be searching for surface clues that reflect the inner state.

The look of the tongue and the skin, the sound of the voice, the strength of the twelve pulses of Chinese medicine, the appearance of the urine, will all be significant. So too, at least for the manipulative disciplines, will be the posture and the balance of muscular tensions.

Iridology – the art of judging the condition of individual organs and parts of the body by examining tiny marks in the iris of the patient's eyes – may also be used for diagnosis.

Treatment
There are very many quite separate systems of alternative medicine – each one complete in itself with its own ideology, its own disciplines, its own educational systems and its own devoted practitioners. But only those thought to offer the possibility of practical benefit to sufferers from rheumatic disease are described in the following pages.

Though every system has its own exclusive idea of the human condition, in practice few therapists consider themselves tightly bound by the boundaries of one single discipline. They often combine aspects of several in their courses of treatment. For rheumatic disease, elements of dietary reform and supplements, homeopathic or herbal medicine, manipulation and exercise, as well as pain relief by acupuncture, hypnotherapy and other means, may well play some part.

A therapist can either concentrate just on tackling specific aspects such as chronic pain and joint immobility, or else attempt more profound healing.

But ultimately it is for the patient to decide whether to limit involvement in a therapy just to alleviating the worst symptoms of an ailment. If the condition is really bad enough, it may justify attempting a complete revolution in the sufferer's established pattern of living – in the hope that at least a partial cure will result. But such revolution really does involve drastic change and total commitment, probably for life.

Further Reading

By far the most useful book on alternative therapies is *The Handbook of Complementary Medicine,* written by Stephen Fulder and published by the Oxford University Press.

Though not related specifically to rheumatic disease, this is a most valuable assessment of a large number of what the author prefers to call complementary therapies. Information from The Handbook proved most helpful in the preparation of parts of this volume.

Another general book on the full range of alternative therapies is *The Alternative Health Guide* by Brian Inglis and Ruth West, published by Mermaid Books.

Naturopathy and Nutritional Therapy

This is a large and complex subject, containing many variations of both theory and treatment. It is, however, possible to set out some fundamental principles.

Self-healing

The first is that, just as the body has the capacity to renew its own cells, heal cuts and mend broken bones, it also has the power to heal itself.

This capacity for self-healing, this inner vitality, can only be stimulated by natural means. These include exercise and fresh air, relaxation of mental stress, the adoption of a natural wholefood diet and the taking of nutritional supplements of a non-toxic nature.

Health

The state of good health means more than simple absence from illness. It exists when body, mind and the environment are in full natural harmony. Disobedience of nature's laws leads inevitably to disease.

Response to Attack

The body and mind respond to attack, physical or emotional, in three distinct phases – alarm, resistance and exhaustion. In the initial alarm stage, the reaction is one of pain, shock or inflammation as appropriate. The resistance stage starts when body and mind begin to adapt in order to resist the trauma – for example by the stiffening of an arthritic joint to prevent damage. The final stage comes when the patient's resistance can no longer cope with what is going on, causing degeneration or collapse.

The concept of a three-staged response is of practical significance during the course of treatment. When the healing process starts (after the collapse condition), mind and body revert to the earlier phases in turn – often causing the temporary flare-up of symptoms commonly described as the healing crisis.

Disease

All forms of illness are due to a common cause. This is the presence in the body of poisonous substances accumulated through living in defiance of natural laws. The toxins derive from harmful foods and pollution and are influenced by hereditary factors. They must be driven out of the body before self-healing can start.

To most naturopaths, the symptoms of disease are the body's sign that it is being poisoned and also evidence of its desperate attempt to eliminate those poisons. Suppressing the symptoms, as in conventional medicine, merely drives them underground to reappear another day in another form.

It is often pointed out, for example, that though treatment with antibiotics will most efficiently destroy the bacteria that have invaded the body, they do nothing to tackle the root cause of the ailment. Unless attended to, this is sure to manifest itself later in a more serious illness.

Diagnosis

Diagnosis on naturopathic principles follows closely that already described in earlier chapters for other forms of alternative medicine.

The patient is seen as a single entity, body and mind. It is he or she who is diagnosed and not just the symptoms of the particular ailment – though these are important too. The therapist will attempt to build up a complete picture of the patient's lifestyle and nutritional condition. An assessment will be made of what has gone wrong, how remaining powers of resistance may best be mobilised and the best methods of so doing.

Most of the standard medical tests, such as the taking of blood pressure, will feature in the diagnosis. And several techniques unacceptable to conventional medicine may be included as well.

Among these is Iridology, first discovered by a German priest who noticed that a blemish appeared in the eye of his pet owl just after it broke a leg; and that the blemish gradually diminished as the leg mended. That initial observation has been developed into a system by means of which the condition of various parts of the body may be learned by studying corresponding areas on the iris of the patient's eye.

Another method sometimes employed is the determination of a patient's nutritional levels, toxic substances and food allergies by means of analysis of samples of hair.

Nourishment   Running parallel with the belief in the cumulatively poisonous effect of eating the wrong foods, and abusing body and mind with unnatural practices (like smoking) and high emotional stress, is the notion that many human beings in modern society are undernourished.

To support this, figures are sometimes quoted comparing modern food to that eaten by primitive man.

Early man's diet appears to have been ten times richer in vitamin C than that of his modern counterpart. The meat from today's farmed animals has eight times more fat than that of wild animals; and it lacks what is now thought to be one of the essential fatty acids (still to be found in some fish). The ratio of polysaturated fat to polyunsaturated fat has also increased by a factor of three. The use of pesticides, artificial fertilisers and food preservatives adds traces of a number of unwelcome chemicals to much contemporary food.

Many of these ideas, such as the desirability of reducing the intake of animal fats, the use of fish oil supplements and the undesirability of chemical additives have already found their way into conventional medical thinking for the prevention of disease.

Other theories, concerning the use of massive doses of vitamins and certain minerals, are still treated with suspicion by conventional medical opinion. It is claimed, though, that there is increasing evidence to support the effectiveness of at least some of them, as well as the belief that arthritis sufferers are deficient in certain key substances.

Nutritional Therapy

The entire field of nutritional therapy has grown by leaps and bounds during the past few years. There is now a considerable literature on the subject, far exceeding that of its parent therapy – naturopathy. However, despite the quantity and complexity of the work being done, nutritional therapy is regarded as being so closely allied to naturopathy that they have been grouped together for the purposes of this book.

Treatment in General

Though in essence very similar, courses of treatment take almost as many different forms as there are naturopaths,

They are based on returning the patient to a state of living in harmony with nature, in which mind and body will best be able to heal themselves.

Elimination from the body of accumulated toxins is usually the first step. This is followed by a strict dietary regime and with supplements to correct nutritional deficiencies.

Exercise, fresh air and relief from emotional stress are essential accompaniments of treatment. Hydrotherapy, osteopathy, chiropractic and acupuncture are very often used in addition.

Various specialised clinics offer residential courses of treatment employing nature cure. Supervised by skilled naturopaths, they often produce good results for those who can afford them.

Unfortunately, in recent years, many such clinics have attracted patients interested primarily in losing weight. Known as health farms, they are mostly very luxurious and expensive. One of the better establishments, offering serious treatment at more moderate cost, is the Tyringham Clinic, Tyringham, Newport Pagnel, Beds. (tel. 0908 610450).

Elimination of Toxins

According to naturopathic theory, the typical modern diet contains far too much red meat, white bread, sugar and preserved foods – all of which leave residues of toxic waste in the body.

The first step in naturopathic treatment, therefore, is to eliminate these poisons.

Fasting for several days is a time-honoured method of ridding the body of unwanted waste products. This is employed to cleanse the system at the start of treatment and periodically after that. Total abstinence during a fast is now often modified to the extent that a single food is permitted – oranges or grapes, for example.

The typical headache, bad breath and thick tongue experienced during the first two or three days of a fast are considered a healthy sign and attributed to the body's throwing off poisons.

The bowels are heavily featured in all naturopathic treatment, especially for rheumatic disease. It is believed that all sufferers from arthritis are constipated to some degree, even if they do have regular bowel movements.

Some therapists think that a slower than desirable process of elimination through the bowels causes toxins to penetrate the wall of the large intestine (the colon) and enter the bloodstream, poisoning the body. Great stress was once put on frequent enemas and the use of laxatives to help purify the system. Mercifully though, this attitude is now sometimes modified in favour of gentler methods.

Apart from the lungs, the other main agent for eliminating toxins from the body is the skin. Bathing in water mixed with Epsom salts is often prescribed. So too are mud baths, mineral baths, steam baths, etc. Another self-help technique favoured is the regular brushing of the skin in a special way in order to stimulate it to expel toxins. Fevers may be induced artificially for this same purpose.

As unimpeded circulation of the blood is also thought necessary for full de-toxification of the system, restrictions caused by muscular tensions are sought out and cleared by massage and other forms of manipulation.

Stress

It is axiomatic that mind and body are inextricably linked. The relief of emotional stress, therefore, is a most important aim of treatment. Stress counselling is recommended, either by the naturopath or by a psychotherapist.

Diet and Supplements

The essential feature is a change to a well-balanced wholefood diet, rich in fibre. Red meat, white bread, sugar and all refined or preserved foods are forbidden. So too is alcohol, tea and coffee. The use of salt is kept to the very minimum.

Vitamin and mineral supplements are given, sometimes in very large doses, to rectify perceived deficiencies. Precisely what supplements are prescribed is a large and complex subject, not covered in this general survey. The interested reader is referred to the many specialised books available on the topic.

Rheumatism and Arthritis

The firm belief is that rheumatic disease is caused by faulty diet. It may also be encouraged by other mental and physical abuse and by hereditary factors.

Naturopaths accept that harmful remnants of food (mostly acidic) remain in the body, where they cannot be neutralised fully by alkaline elements because of deficiencies in modern methods of refining and cooking food.

Also, lack of fibre in many modern diets inhibits the prompt and thorough elimination of these toxins. They accumulate on the muscles and bones, and in the joints, giving rise to the symptoms of arthritis and rheumatism.

In addition, it is thought that most sufferers from arthritis are deficient in certain key vitamins and minerals.

Treatment for arthritis and rheumatism, therefore, is very little different from the standard procedures outlined above.

Elimination and fasting are the invariable first steps, followed by change of diet, dietary supplements, skin treatments, hydrotherapy, exercise, massage, manipulation, acupuncture and so on, as appropriate. It must be remembered that it is the patient who is diagnosed and treated, not just the symptoms; and so treatment will vary for each individual.

Personal Programmes of Cure

At any one time, bookshops stock books written by different people who have cured themselves of arthritis by natural means and wish to share the good news of their achievement. Books are also available on recommended programmes of self-help, written by practitioners of nature cure.

Three of the ones most readily available when this chapter was being written, selected almost at random, are mentioned below as typical examples of what can be done. There are many others.

Curing Arthritis The Drug-Free Way by Margaret Hills S.R.N., published by Sheldon Press, London.

In this book, Margaret Hills tells how she managed to cure herself of crippling arthritis by means of her own version of the nature cure. She progressed from a state of disability to lead a useful, active life and now runs her own arthritis clinic in Coventry.

Nurse Hills, who also claims to have healing powers, prescribes the natural, high-fibre diet outlined above – but with variations. In her method, stress is placed on the acidic nature of toxins accumulated in the body; and, for example, all citrus fruit is banned because of its acidic nature.

Dietary supplementation is considered necessary and Nurse Hills gives her patients multi-vitamin pills, but not the massive doses recommended by some, as well as other supplements.

In addition to her version of the natural diet, Margaret Hills insists on her patients also taking regularly the three additional products that worked so well in her own case. These are cider vinegar (acidic!), honey and black molasses. She gives full explanations of the benefit to be derived from regular doses of each of these substances.

Like all naturopaths, Nurse Hills believes in the importance of exercise and in methods of reducing stress.

She does not endorse the purging insisted on by some; but concentrates rather on Epsom Salt bathing to facilitate elimination of toxins through the skin.

Triumph Over Arthritis by Anna H. Scott, published by Hale and Iremonger of Sydney, Australia.

This is only one of the many books on arthritis published in Australia. In it, Anna Scott tells how she rose above the despair caused by the extreme disability to which she had been reduced by arthritis and, influenced by a naturopath, cured herself by natural means.

She started by drinking vast quantities of carrot juice and apple juice and then proceeded, by use of the kind of natural diet described above, to rid her body of toxins and replace them with the nourishment she so badly needed.

Relaxation and the relief of tension also helped in her cure, as did exercise and the dietary supplements taken on the advice of her nature cure practitioner. The results achieved appear remarkable; and it must be said that Anna Scott's account of her journey from sickness to health seems to carry an unmistakable stamp of authenticity.

The larger part of the book is devoted to separate explanations of the many different alternative therapies thought to be of benefit to sufferers from arthritis, each written by a qualified practitioner in the particular subject.

Arthritis by Leon Chaitow, published by Thorsons, London.

Leon Chaitow, a well-known naturopath, examines the causes of arthritis and describes a programme of self-help therapy for it, based on natural treatments without the use of drugs.

Mr Chaitow's recommended methods include stretching exercises, hydrotherapy, massage, muscle energy technique, herbal remedies and nutritional advice. The author also provides guidance on dealing with stress and other emotional factors. Much of this has already been described earlier in this chapter and will not be repeated here.

Like some other naturopaths, the author very much believes in the method of skin friction – brushing the skin in a certain sequence – as a very effective way of accelerating the removal of toxins through the skin and also to enhance the lymphatic drainage of body tissues.

On the nutritional side, Chaitow endorses the view that acidic citrus fruit should be eaten sparingly if at all. Bowel health is important. Supplements such as vitamins and the mineral selenium are recommended.

In his section on bowel health, the author warns that man is not well adapted to digesting grains and dairy food, which are best avoided by many who cannot tolerate them.

Natural remedies recommended include an extract of New Zealand green-lipped mussels, and Squalene which is an extract of deep-sea sharks. Beneficial herbs include the African devil's claw, as well as alfalfa and comfrey root.

Copper Bracelets

This is a highly controversial subject. Many thousands of people wear copper bracelets against arthritis and a large number of these believe they are of use. Sceptics, on the other hand, dismiss bracelets as no more than absurd superstition.

A theory has recently emerged that the bodies of sufferers from arthritis require far more copper than those of other people; and that the bracelets work because copper from them is absorbed into the body through the skin of the wrist.

A number of tests have been carried out on this idea; and it is claimed that the results are encouraging if inconclusive.

All, however, agree that copper bracelets cannot possibly do any harm. It will be interesting to see whether this old folk remedy will eventually be justified by medical science. Far stranger things have happened!

A Useful Organisation

The *Arthritic Association* was founded in 1942 by a group of forty-two people who had one thing in common – they had all recovered from arthritis.

It developed considerably during the following fifty years and now provides members with a programme of home treatment, dietary guidance, homeopathic, herbal, vitamin and mineral tablets at reduced cost, as well as the services of a consultant in London and Eastbourne for private consultation and treatment. It also issues a magazine twice a year, which helps to keep members in touch.

The methods of treatment recommended are essentially naturopathic, but with the addition of homeopathic remedies.

The founder of the Arthritic Association firmly believed that arthritis begins in the bowel and is due to incorrect diet causing a deficiency of potassium in the blood.

The Association claims to have helped many thousands of people regain freedom of movement, freedom from pain and a healthier life. Quoting from one of its publications, *We who were crippled can now walk!*

Membership particulars may be obtained from The Arthritic Association, 1 Park View, 6 Park Avenue, Eastbourne, East Sussex BN22 9QN.

Professional Association

British Naturopathic and Osteopathic Association, 6 Netherhall Gardens, London NW3 5RR. Telephone: 071 435 8728.

The Association is open to graduates of the British School of Naturopathy and Osteopathy and others suitably qualified.

There are over 200 naturopaths in practice in the U.K. Members use the letters M.B.N.O.A. after their names.

Further Reading

Overcoming Arthritis and Rheumatic Diseases by Max Warmbrand. Published by Bachman and Turner, London.

Everybody's Guide to Nature Cure by Harry Benjamin. Published by Thorsons.

This classic was first published in 1936 and has been reprinted many times. It now seems rather dated; but nevertheless presents an excellent picture of the supremely confident naturopathic approach to the problems of illness.

Acupuncture and Traditional Chinese Medicine

History

Traditional Chinese medicine dates back in time to the Stone Age. Its leading text was written well over two thousand years ago and its practice had already been codified substantially by the end of the sixth century.

It is still widely used in China, especially in country districts where it is represented alongside conventional Western medicine in many hospitals. Taiwan and Hong Kong are other important centres of this method of treatment. Traditional Chinese medicine is also taught and practised in this country by devoted therapists.

Chinese medicine is a self-contained system. It is used to maintain good health, detect the early stages of illness and treat sickness – all by combinations of exercise, massage, acupuncture, diet and herbs.

Acupuncture caught the imagination of doctors and public in the West in the 1970s, when surgeons in China successfully demonstrated how, with its use, operations can be performed without anaesthetics.

The actual technique of acupuncture, divorced from its roots in Chinese medicine, is now accepted by the medical profession as a complementary therapy for pain relief. Such treatment is available in some of the pain clinics run by the National Health Service; but this use is, of course, quite different from that of employing acupuncture as a component of traditional Chinese medicine.

Western doctors further developed the technique of acupuncture by adding modern methods to the traditional Chinese ones; and these have had influence in China itself.

Again, not directly related to traditional Chinese theory, a French doctor discovered a large number of reflex points on the ear which are related to other parts of the body. These may also be stimulated by acupuncture needles; and this therapy, further developed, is also in use today.

The Basic Principle

All life, including human life, is animated by a form of vital energy which the Chinese call *Chi*.

This energy flows though the body along a network of channels called *meridians,* parts of which pass over its surface.

The flow of chi is free and balanced in a healthy body. A disturbed flow indicates disease.

Meridians

Each of the twelve main meridians, along which the vital energy flows, is connected to an organ of the body. There are also two additional meridians.

Meridians pass over the surface of the body and deep inside it. For example, the meridian of the large intestine (the colon) runs inside the body from the intestine to the nose. It then continues along the surface, over the neck and shoulder and down the arm to the tip of the index finger.

Each of the twelve main meridians has its own pulse, which is an important factor in diagnosis.

The existence of actual physical meridians, as visualised by the Chinese therapists, is denied by Western medical scientists; but they have not yet succeeded in finding an acceptable alternative explanation for the associated phenomena.

Yin and Yang

The flow of chi along the meridians is activated by the two opposing forces of *Yin* and *Yang,* between which the vital energy is in constant movement.

Yin is the male force, active and positive. Yang is its female counterpart, passive and negative. There is continuous interaction between the yin and yang forces in the body; and for health, these must be finely balanced.

Some organs and connecting meridians, such as heart, liver and kidneys, are associated with yin; and others, such as stomach, bladder and intestines, with yang.

Health

In the state of good health, chi flows freely throughout the body in a balanced manner. Chinese practitioners prescribe daily exercises, massage, herbal remedies and close attention to diet in order to strengthen the flow of chi and prevent disease.

Sickness

Disturbance to the flow of vital energy along the meridians causes sickness.

This can happen because of a variety of factors, internal and external. The internal factors include heredity, emotional stress and various abuses of the body such as heavy smoking or excessive eating or drinking.

Somewhat surprisingly to a Western observer, changes in climatic conditions loom very large in the list of external factors, which also include more obvious causes like shock.

It is the aim of Chinese practitioners to detect and then correct subtle changes in the flow of chi before the onset of a resulting illness. When disease does occur, they will attempt to cure it by similar means.

Acupuncture Points

Several individual points have been identified along the path of each meridian at which the flow of chi may be adjusted in different ways. These are called the acupuncture points.

Intervention is effected by the use of fine needles at the acupuncture points *(acupuncture)*. Heat may also be applied to them *(moxibustion)*, or they may be pressed and massaged by the fingers *(acupressure)*. More modern means, such as electrical impulses, ultrasonic waves or laser beams, may also be used to stimulate the flow of energy at the acupuncture points.

Acupuncture

The actual process of acupuncture consists of pushing fine steel needles though the skin at the particular acupuncture points indicated by diagnosis. This is done to relieve pain or to treat disease by correcting the flow of chi in the meridians.

The needles are rotated or otherwise manipulated by the therapist to produce the desired effect. In some cases, a small cone of moxa (dried mugwort) may also be placed on the end of the needle and slowly burned to deliver heat to the acupuncture point in order to strengthen the flow of chi. The same effect is sometimes obtained by applying a small electric current to the needle.

Only very slight pricks are felt as the needles go in; and some patients feel nothing at all. There may be an almost painful or numbing sensation as energy flow along the meridians is stimulated. It must be stressed, though, that acupuncture does not hurt and is a far from unpleasant experience.

As mentioned above, some of the more modern variations of technique avoid penetrating the skin altogether. In them, needles are replaced by laser beams or other devices to stimulate the acupuncture points in similar manner.

Though totally rejecting the underlying theories of traditional Chinese medicine, conventional doctors now accept that acupuncture works – to some extent at least – and they are still trying to find a satisfactory explanation for its effects.

Also, there can be little doubt that the acupuncture points really do exist, for they have been shown to be places on the skin of particularly low electrical resistance. In fact, changes in resistance of acupuncture points along particular meridians have, in some tests, been shown to be related directly to the particular organ to which they are connected.

After treatment, patients often experience an exhilarating sense of well-being but they may also feel slightly dizzy or sleepy. These feelings soon disappear.

Diagnosis   Diagnosis is subtle and complex. The approach is holistic, in that all parts of the body and mind are inter-dependent; and changes to one part will always affect others in some way. The final diagnosis will not be clear-cut, as in Western medicine, for there are few exact answers in the Chinese tradition.

The therapist will first try to build up a complete picture of the patient, including details of heredity, medical history, personality, likes and dislikes, etc. The charting of emotional patterns is an essential part of this process.

The practitioner will then attempt to assess the extent to which the flow of chi has been interrupted and its balance disturbed. For this, the traditional techniques of listening, smelling, looking, asking and touching will be used.

The quality (not the rate, as in conventional medicine) of the pulse on each of the twelve meridians will be examined in detail. This is a highly skilled operation and is considered most important. There are no fewer than twenty-eight different qualities that can be assigned to each pulse.

The state of the tongue is another leading indicator. So too will close attention be given to the appearance and feel of the skin, to the breathing, to the eyes, the voice and the urine. Blood pressure may also be taken and the abdomen palpated.

Treatment

Acupuncture, to correct imbalances between yin and yang in the flow of vital energy through the body, looms large in traditional treatment of disease. But other methods, such as diet and the administration of complex mixtures of herbs, are also used in conjunction with it. There are over one hundred different herbs in use for the treatment of arthritis alone.

A temporary flare-up of symptoms during treatment, or rashes on the skin, are interpreted as a sign that the cure is working. The disturbance soon subsides and there are no other ill effects.

Arthritis and Rheumatism

According to the theory of traditional Chinese medicine, arthritis is caused by obstruction of the circulation of chi, vital energy, in the body.

The factors causing this state, known as the Bi Syndrome, are associated with the conditions of wind, hot, cold and damp. Each of the many kinds of arthritis, identified by conventional Western medicine, finds its place under one or more of these traditional Chinese categories.

Treatment by acupuncture and by subtle mixtures of special herbs is intended to relieve symptoms and, more important, to remove the root causes of the arthritis.

It cannot regenerate destroyed or badly damaged joints. But in cases where serious permanent damage has not yet occurred, it is claimed that a complete cure can sometimes be achieved.

At the very least, acupuncture has often proved remarkably effective in suppressing pain, restoring joint mobility and reducing inflammation. Most certainly, Chinese medicine does not cause any of the harmful side-effects experienced as the result of prolonged drug-taking.

Complementary Therapy

In its use as a pain reliever, without any of the aims or trappings of Chinese medicine, acupuncture is now considered as a complementary therapy to conventional medical treatment.

**Useful
Organisations**

It should be noted that there are many doubtful schools and organisations promoting some kind of acupuncture and that seemingly impressive strings of qualifications may not always amount to very much.

Among the most reputable organisations are the following:

International College of Oriental Medicine, Green Hedges Avenue, East Grinstead, Sussex RH19 1DZ. Tel. 0342 313106

This is reputed to be one of the most thorough schools of Chinese medicine in the West. It also gives grounding in conventional medicine.

It maintains the *Register of Traditional Chinese Medicine* at 19 Trinity Road, London N2 8JJ. Tel. 081 883 8431. The Register includes between fifty and one hundred full members in practice in the U.K. They are entitled to use the letters M.R.T.C.M. after their names.

College of Traditional Chinese Acupuncture, Tao House, Queensway, Leamington Spa, Warwickshire CV31 3LZ. Tel. 0926 422 121.

This provides rather similar but shorter courses to those of the International College listed above. Its associated *Traditional Acupuncture Society* maintains a register of full members at 1 The Ridgeway, Stratford upon Avon, Warwickshire CV37 9JL. Tel. 0789 298 798.

Full members use the letters M.T.Ac.S or F.T.Ac.S. after their names.

British College of Acupuncture, Old Royal Free School of Medicine, 8 Hunter Street, London WC1N 1BN. Tel. 071 833 8164.

This aims to combine traditional acupuncture with a conventional Western medical approach. Its courses are shorter than those of the two colleges named above and less emphasis is given to underlying theory.

The *British Acupuncture Association and Register,* at the same address, is the associated professional organisation.

It maintains a register of over two hundred members in practice in the U.K.

Members and Fellows use the letters M.B.Ac.A. and F.B.Ac.A. after their names. Associate members, with no orthodox medical training, use the letters A.M.B.Ac.A.

Acupressure

Theory and Practice

This is a simplified form of acupuncture without needles. In it, the acupuncture points are stimulated by simply pressing them with the fingers. It is known in America as G-Jo.

Its theory and practice are based on the same principles of traditional Chinese medicine described in the last chapter. Indeed, acupressure is sometimes used by therapists in preference to acupuncture for the treatment of young children.

Like acupuncture, acupressure may be employed as a natural aid to conventional medical treatment – for it can help to reduce pain, promote relaxation and encourage healing. When used in this limited way, belief or otherwise in the principles of traditional Chinese medicine becomes less important. What matters is that the therapy does seem to work.

In fact acupressure, being less precise and less powerful than acupuncture, may well be more suited to the role of a subsidiary self-help programme of relief than as a complete therapy for the treatment of rheumatic disease.

Self-help Programmes

Several practitioners have developed programmes of self-help, using acupressure and related exercises. The techniques are relatively easy to learn, especially if one or two lessons can first be taken with an expert therapist.

For arthritis and rheumatism, there are several programmes available.

One programme is described in *The Natural Healer's Acupressure Handbook*, Volumes 1 and 2, written by Michael Bate and published by Routledge and Kegan Paul.

The first volume deals with the basic technique for relieving pain, relaxing tense muscles and encouraging circulation by a deep digging or goading type of pressure on selected acupuncture points. The author describes this as *fingertip aspirin*. In the second volume, the method of locating and treating the true causes of the disease is described in a technique called Advanced G-Jo.

Another of the better programmes, readily available in bookshops, was also devised in America. This is very clearly set out and explained in a book entitled *Arthritis Relief at your Fingertips*, written by Michael Reed Gach and published by Judy Piatkus (Publishers) Ltd

It is designed as a self-help programme to relieve pain and inflammation, restore flexibility to stiff joints and decrease stress. No claim is made for it as a complete therapy or cure in itself; but its author does hold out the hope that, by achieving a general improvement, the need to take harmful drugs will be reduced.

Michael Gach claims that a large number of people have been helped by his programme. He points out that, though immediate relief is felt as soon as pressure is applied to the indicated acupuncture points, this is temporary. The programme must be followed daily for about six months before a measurable result can be expected.

Reactions to Treatment

A reaction is usually experienced after sessions of acupressure. There may be a feeling of warmth or a flush of perspiration on the forehead or neck. There may also be deep relaxation and sometimes fleeting sensations of queasiness, lightheadedness or even nausea.

During deep treatment for arthritis, a flare up of the condition may be expected as the healing process starts; and this may well be accompanied by general aches and pains or emotional distress.

The Time Factor

Practitioners urge patience and perseverance. They say, quite rightly, that one cannot expect to cure in days conditions that it has taken years or even decades to create.

Shiatsu

Theory and Practice

Shiatsu was developed fully in Japan fifty or so years ago. It is so similar to acupressure that both are often considered parts of the same therapy. The difference is that Shiatsu uses massage as well as pressure to obtain its effects.

Firmly based on the principles of traditional Chinese medicine, described in an earlier chapter, diagnosis and treatment follow precisely the same pattern. But in Shiatsu, the acupuncture needles of Chinese therapy are replaced by finger pressure and a complex system of massage.

Shiatsu is, by its very nature, not so precise or powerful as acupuncture and therefore requires less knowledge for its use. It is employed widely in Japan to maintain health, detect early signs of illness and treat disease. Interestingly, in Japan, it was one of the occupations traditionally open to the blind.

Uses

The therapy is insufficiently established in this country to be administered as a complete treatment for arthritis, except perhaps by one or two practitioners. It may however be used as a complementary therapy to full treatment by another system of alternative medicine or by conventional medicine.

Depending on the knowledge and skill of the therapist, Shiatsu can be very effective in reducing pain and inflammation, helping to restore the mobility of stiff joints, bringing about a diminution of stress and a general improvement of the condition.

Treatment

A session with a therapist consists of the application of pressure to the acupuncture points, coupled with a complicated system of massaging the points and the meridians on which they are situated.

Therapists are taught to apply sufficient pressure to reach the borderline between pleasure and pain – but not to cross it. So, though perhaps very slightly painful at times, the total experience is said to be pleasurable.

Useful Address

The Shiatsu Society, 14 Oakdene Road Redhill RH1 6BT, tel. 0737 767896, maintains a list of therapists and teachers active in this country.

Reflexology

Origins and Modern Use

This is a very old form of traditional Chinese medicine, also practised in ancient Egypt.

It was rediscovered by an American surgeon, who managed to perform operations on the ear without anaesthetic simply by applying pressure to the sole of the foot just behind the second toe.

The technique was introduced into this country in the 1960s. It is a suitable therapy for those with rheumatism or arthritis of various kinds, including chronic back pain.

Underlying Theory

Like other forms of Chinese medicine, reflexology depends on the theory of the body's vital energy. Good health is enjoyed when this flows freely. Disease results from its being impeded. True cure can only be achieved through the body's own power of self-healing.

The actual therapy depends on the belief that every part of the body is connected by energy pathways, all of which terminate in the feet, hands and head.

Reflex points for all organs and parts of the body are located in the feet, with each foot representing its own side of the body. Corresponding points exist in the hands, though these are not used in the therapy.

Practice

In consequence, massage of a part of the foot will have an effect in the distant region corresponding to it. Circulation of the blood in that area will be improved and muscular tensions relaxed. Vital energy will be stimulated at the same time, enabling the healing process to start.

Trouble in one part of the body will also be reflected by tenderness at its corresponding reflex point in the foot. This will became a source of pain under massage, when it may feel as if the therapist is pressing a sharp finger nail into the skin.

Sometimes a tiny deposit or lump will also be found just under the skin at a reflex point. This can be broken up by massage, after which it will dissolve.

In keeping with the principles of holistic medicine, the entire body is treated by foot massage at each session, and not just the troubled part.

Results

Therapists warn that results cannot be expected at once and that it may take several months before measurable improvement is achieved.

A healing crisis may occur as the cure begins to take effect and the body expels its accumulated toxins. This may take the form of a skin rash, a mild fever or other symptoms.

Homeopathy

History

Though the principles of homeopathy were recognised by the ancient Greeks, as well as in sixteenth century Europe, a method of treatment employing them was first developed in Germany. Dr. Samuel Hahnemann, a respected Medical Officer of Health, published the first book on the subject in 1811. Hahnemann's system of cure was further developed after his death and that process continues.

The first homeopathic hospital in this country was opened in Great Ormond Street, London, in 1844; and only ten years later it was claimed that its mortality rates were considerably lower than for those for all other London hospitals. There are now similar hospitals in Glasgow, Bristol, Tunbridge Wells and Liverpool. They all provide in-patient and out-patient treatment within the National Health Service.

Homeopathy almost died out after the discovery of penicillin, antibiotics and the other wonder drugs earlier this century. But with the waning of confidence in some drugs, interest in homeopathy has sharply revived.

Some homeopaths first train as doctors; and indeed the qualification for sitting the examination for full membership of the Faculty of Homeopathy is an orthodox medical degree. Many other homeopathic practitioners are not medical doctors, but are simply trained in their own discipline.

Though bitterly opposed by the medical profession as a whole, homeopathy has attained a certain respectability because the Queen and other members of the royal family acknowledge being treated regularly by this method. Homeopathy is more popular on the continent, especially in France and Germany. In France, for example, it has been estimated that about one prescription in four, dispensed by the country's pharmacists, is homeopathic.

Principles Hahnemann based his methods on the principle that *like is cured by like* – a preparation that *causes* certain symptoms in a healthy person will actually *cure* those same symptoms when given to a sick person. The same kind of idea is, of course, used by conventional doctors in vaccination.

Hahnemann's really amazing discovery was that, provided his remedies were violently shaken when being diluted, the smaller the dose administered the greater its effect. In fact, the most potent doses of homeopathic medicine prescribed are diluted many millions of times.

Scientists are still trying to come up with a convincing explanation for this extraordinary phenomenon; and sceptics refuse to believe that such dilutions – often containing one or two molecules, at most, of the original substance – can possibly work.

Vital Force The belief underlying homeopathic medicine is that human beings are animated by a form of energy called the vital force.

All cells in the human body, from those of the main organs to those of the skin, are in a constant state of self-renewal. The vital force controls this function as well as the body's power of self-healing, if indeed there is any difference between them. Disturbance to the vital force causes sickness. When it is overwhelmed by disturbances and can no longer cope with them, the vital force then produces the symptoms of disease. Symptoms therefore are *not* the true disease, but merely signs of the body's reaction to a deeper cause.

Healing can only be achieved by the body itself, using its own resources; and the homeopath's task is to stimulate the power of self-healing.

According to theory, there is no incurable disease but only incurable people. When a patient's power of self-healing has been too badly eroded by steroids, prolonged drug treatment, radiation or other destructive processes, a cure becomes very much more difficult if not impossible.

Diagnosis and Treatment

In homeopathic treatment, the self-healing power of the body's vital force is stimulated by the administration of minute doses of a substance that will produce in a healthy person symptoms similar to those of the disease. For example, the symptoms of gastroenteritis are so alike those of arsenic poisoning that minute doses of arsenic are effective in curing gastroenteritis.

Of course it is more complicated than that. The homeopath needs to build up a complete picture of the patient and symptoms before attempting to match those to the single remedy ideal for treatment.

This perfect matching of patient with remedy is so important that, in most cases, only a single remedy will be tried at any one time. A combination of several is unusual and probably will not work.

Rheumatism and Arthritis

Rheumatic disease, believed to be triggered partly by hereditary factors, is thought to be a symptom of the reduced capacity of the body to eliminate accumulations of toxic substances.

In arthritis, for example, these poisons are deposited in the joints where they typically give rise to deterioration and inflammation.

Homeopathic treatment for arthritis, therefore, concentrates first on expelling the toxins accumulated in the joints. It then seeks to eliminate them from the body by stimulating the kidneys and lymphatic drainage. The liver is stimulated at the same time to purify the blood and improve its circulation, as well as strengthening the digestion to reduce any further build-up of poisons.

In diagnosis, all aspects of the patient and primary and secondary symptoms are studied to build up a complete picture to which a homeopathic remedy can then be matched.

This includes details of personality traits, likes and dislikes, reaction to cold and heat, physical appearance, etc. The patient's emotional history is an essential part of such assessment.

The remedies, always given in tiny doses, are almost free from risk.

Response to Treatment

Some initial vomiting or diarrhea may be experienced as the body starts to eliminate its toxins; and this is interpreted as a sign that the healing process has started. In classic homeopathic theory, symptoms of a disease will move outwards from their source as healing progresses. Eventually they will pass to the surface of the skin, which may break out in rashes or spasms of itching.

Treatment of Symptoms

Homeopathic treatment for rheumatic disease concentrates on removing its root cause and does not directly address its symptoms. A homeopathic doctor will probably recommend other therapists who will also be able to help with massage and exercise, diet, acupuncture and other natural means.

Useful Organisations

The Faculty of Homeopathy, The Royal London Homeopathic Hospital, Great Ormond Street, London WC1 3HR. Tel. 071 837 3091.

Full membership is open only to those with a medical degree. There are well over three hundred full members in practice in the U.K. They use the letters M.F.Hom. after their names.

The Society of Homeopaths Ltd, 2 Artizan Road, Northampton NN1 4HU. Tel. 0604 21400.

Full membership is granted after approval by an examinations committee. There are fewer than one hundred full members in practice in the U.K. They use the letters R.S.Hom. after their names.

British Homeopathic Association, 27a Devonshire Street, London W1N 1RJ. Tel. 071 935 2163.

This is a major support and information organisation with over five thousand members.

Herbalism, Aromatherapy and Bach Flower Therapy

History

The use of naturally grown herbs to treat disease must be the very first form of medical science in history. It is scientific in that the efficacy of each particular herb has been established by trial and error over hundreds if not thousands of years.

There are well over one hundred qualified medical herbalists in practice in this country. Some adopt the alternative approach to healing, whilst others incline to a more conventional medical viewpoint.

Herbal remedies are an essential component of traditional Chinese medicine. They are often used by naturopaths, osteopaths and other alternative practitioners in conjunction with their own therapies. A particular Chinese herb has just become available by prescription in the National Health Service.

Basic Principles

There is no central organisation to lay down basic beliefs, for herbal medicine has long been practised all over the world in a variety of ways.

It is probably fair to assert that most herbalists support the idea that a form of vital energy permeates each human being, and that this is responsible for the body's resistance to attack and for its powers of self-healing and regeneration.

Disease is seen as a sign of some deep disturbance of this vital energy, manifesting itself in the observed symptoms. Treatment therefore is directed at the underlying cause as well as at the symptoms themselves.

The above concepts are only mentioned here in barest outline as they have already been described in more detail in earlier chapters devoted to other systems of alternative medicine.

It is not really understood why herbs are found to be so much more effective than drugs – which, after all, mostly started as synthetic imitations of naturally occurring plant drugs – nor why an extract of the active element in a herb should be inferior to the whole herb. One possible explanation offered is that nature endows plants with a certain balance which is lost if the whole plant is not used.

Diagnosis and Herbal Treatment

Diagnosis follows closely along the holistic lines already discussed elsewhere in this book. Many herbal practitioners also use the tools of conventional doctors to aid diagnosis.

Herbs are employed in many different ways. They can adjust and restore normality to disturbed bodily functions, sometimes acting more like special foods than medicines. They can also help to trigger required responses in particular areas. Some herbs have healing properties of their own.

Another most important range of uses is in stimulating those processes which eliminate toxins from the body, such as circulation of the blood and drainage of the tissues. Sweat glands, kidneys, lungs and bowels are the key organs in this work.

The list of uses for medicinal herbs continues, seemingly without limit. Many different herbs will be employed in the treatment of each patient and their number and composition will vary as the cure progresses.

Rheumatic Disease

Herbal practitioners, in common with most other alternative therapists, attribute rheumatic disease to an excessive accumulation of toxic waste products in the body.

The body's failure to eliminate these poisons, and cope with the situation in general, may be due to faulty diet, lack of fresh air and exercise, emotional strain or other abuses like heavy smoking and drinking.

The casting out of toxins and the substitution of a healthy diet are the essential components of all treatment. Building up the body's powers of resistance and restoring the balance of vital energy are also aspects of crucial importance.

Where poor bowel movement is thought to be a major source of the problem, causing toxins to be re-absorbed into the bloodstream, the taking of a certain range of herbs is a most efficient method of correction.

Some herbal products are used to purify the blood and others to restore proper circulation to all parts of the body.

Another class of herbs is employed for the quite different task of mobilising the liver and strengthening digestion. This encourages the body's own digestive system to deal with more of the toxins itself, thus reducing the amount left to be disposed of by other means.

Herbs are also used directly to relieve troublesome symptoms. The bark of willow trees, for example, is helpful in reducing the inflammation and swelling associated with rheumatoid arthritis. Claims are made that evening primrose oil has similar effect.

As sufferers from arthritis will probably not seek to depend only on herbal medicine for treatment, and are far more likely to use herbal remedies in conjunction with other therapies, the subject is not discussed further here. However, the range of herbs available, and the claims made for them, make for fascinating reading. Those interested are referred to specialised books on the subject.

Aromatherapy Aromatherapy is a branch of herbal medicine, subject to the same theories of diagnosis and treatment. The technique is useful for the relief of stress-related ailments and is also said to be of some help to sufferers from rheumatism and arthritis.

The therapist employs aromatic essences for treatment. These are highly concentrated essential oils derived from herbs, flowers, spices and resins. There are over two hundred such oils available, thus allowing a very large number of different combinations to be used as appropriate.

The oils are usually administered through the skin by massage. They may also be inhaled or applied in creams and lotions.

Though some therapists strongly disapprove, oils may also be administered in tiny doses by mouth. For arthritis, oils such as onion, garlic, juniper, marjoram and lemon may be taken with meals, either on a sugar lump or else diluted in a drink.

Aromatherapy cannot be regarded as a complete treatment for arthritis and practitioners in this country are not yet in a position to undertake such responsibility.

Bach Flower Therapy

Dr Edward Bach, who died in 1936, used the essences of flowers to treat emotional disorder.

His therapy is not intended to deal directly with physical disease, such as arthritis, but concentrates on the states of mind that not only hinder recovery but are a primary cause of sickness.

Thirty-eight wild flowers were selected by Dr Bach to match different negative mental states and these may also be used in combination.

There are very few Bach Flower therapists in practice today. But an explanatory book, advice and the remedies themselves may be obtained from the *Dr. Edward Bach Centre,* Mount Vernon, Sotwell, Oxfordshire OX10 0PZ, telephone 0491 39489. The remedies may also be bought at some Health Food shops.

Useful Address

National Institute of Medical Herbalists Ltd. 9 Palace Gate, Exeter EX1 1JA. Tel. 0392 426022

This is the leading professional institution. Its members are all graduates of *The School of Herbal Medicine,* which runs proper full-time courses in the subject lasting over several years.

Well over one hundred members of the National Institute of Medical Herbalists practice in the U.K. They are entitled to use the letters M.N.I.M.H. after their names.

Mind Therapies

General

The belief that the mind and body function as a single entity, and that changes in one part inevitably involve changes in the other, is a fundamental belief shared by most alternative therapies. This holistic view, in which body and mind are closely intertwined, is also held by many doctors.

Examples of how the mind can affect the body have already been given in the earlier chapters on alternative systems of medicine and will not be repeated here. The reader is referred in particular to pages 61 and 62.

The onset of arthritis is often triggered by acute emotional shock, such as the death of a loved one; and the relief of stress is an important part of most intelligent programmes for treating rheumatic disease, whether by alternative or conventional means.

Mind therapies that deal effectively with the stress factor can therefore be useful in the treatment of rheumatic disease. They may not feature prominently but can be important nevertheless.

Hypnotherapy Hypnosis is one of the few non-conventional therapies to have gained partial recognition by the medical profession – though this was achieved only after a long struggle.

There can be no doubt that the mind is far more open to suggestion from the outside when in a state of hypnosis. It can then perform considerable feats.

For arthritis, the hypnotic state may be induced by skilled therapists for the relief of pain, sometimes with dramatic result. Tests indicate that it can have a more powerful effect than acupuncture or pain-killing drugs. Hypnosis is sometimes used in this way in National Health Service pain clinics.

Hypnosis can also be a very useful tool in the hands of a psychotherapist trying to reduce emotional stress in a patient. After several sessions, the therapist may teach the patient to develop his or her own power of self-hypnosis to enable treatment to be maintained on a continuing basis.

In theory at least, the same technique may be applied to suppress symptoms of arthritis such as inflammation and swelling. The patient can simply be told under hypnosis that his swollen knee, for example, will get better. And sometimes it really will do so – for a while. But as the real cause of the swelling remains untouched, the *cure* is an illusion which will not last for long. It is for this reason that hypnotherapy is seldom used directly for the treatment of rheumatic disease.

Hypnotherapy has another role for those who believe in theories that it is only the body's own vital energy that can bring about a true cure. This is described below.

**Faith
Healing**

If the mind really can influence the body, any method able to stimulate the body's powers of regeneration and self-healing must clearly be of value.

The faith healer first has to gain the total confidence and trust of the patient. Only when this has been accomplished can the healer work directly on the patient's mind to achieve the desired result.

As the mind is at its most receptive to suggestion in the hypnotic state, hypnosis is sometimes used by faith healers in such efforts to assist patients to mobilise their own inner resources and generate the power necessary to heal themselves.

The healing process may also be helped along by many of the methods used in one or more of the other natural therapies; for it must make sense to provide the body with all possible assistance.

**Relaxation,
Yoga and
Meditation**

Relaxation, as a method of controlling and overcoming the emotional stress considered so harmful to sufferers from rheumatic disease, has already been described in the chapter on Conventional Management in Part Three of this book. The reader is referred to page 48 above.

The initial stages of Yoga and Transcendental Meditation achieve very much the same result as Relaxation, which is in fact based on their techniques. In their further stages, they then proceed to deeper levels of consciousness, beyond that achieved by simple Relaxation.

These three very similar alternative methods can be of value in the prevention and treatment of certain kinds of disease. In so far as arthritis and rheumatism sufferers are concerned, a controlled relaxation of mental stress, together with the relief of harmful muscular tension, must be beneficial in all forms of treatment.

**Autogenic
Therapy**

This is a further development of the methods of relaxation and hypnotism to form a separate specialised therapy in its own right.

It is certainly not suitable for all patients. Those selected are trained in a particular method of progressive relaxation, combined with a kind of self-hypnosis.

Once enabled to enter at will into that mental state, the conscious mind can then learn gradually how to control automatic body functions such as heartbeat, muscular tension and skin temperature. This acquired ability can then be used to alleviate some symptoms of illness.

No direct cure of any particular disease is ever attempted. The aim is simply to liberate the body's own flow of vital energies in order to enable self-healing to take place.

Biofeedback Though only indirectly applicable to the problems of rheumatic disease – and then probably just for the relief of stress and muscular tension – a few words on this therapy are included here because of what can be learned from it concerning the influence of mind over body.

The therapy got its initial boost when experimenters successfully demonstrated that laboratory animals can be taught to control functions such as heartbeat, blood pressure and skin temperature.

Human subjects are hooked up to a battery of measuring instruments which will record their brain waves, blood pressure, electrical skin resistance, heartbeat, etc.

They then enter into the same sort of relaxed, almost hypnotic, mental state used in autogenic therapy. There they learn gradually how to control their own body functions, using the instruments to which they are connected to monitor progress. The aim is eventually to acquire sufficient skill and confidence to be able to do without the machines.

Biofeedback stands on an exciting new frontier of learning which is fully scientific. Moreover it is free from all theory deriving from alternative therapy which is unacceptable to traditional medicine. It has yet to be developed into a useful therapy; but this is sure to follow as more research is undertaken into its amazing possibilities.

Psychic and Spiritual Healing

This subject has been left to the last as it is not really a *mind* therapy at all, but rather one of the *spirit*.

Its main branch derives from the special gift possessed by certain individuals, who seem able to transfer a mysterious healing power of their own to others by touch, prayer or other means.

Some alternative therapists claim also to possess this gift of healing. A good example is that of Margaret Hills, whose experience and work are described on page 71 of this book. Nurse Hills discovered her own gift by chance when she happened to touch one of her patients and both then experienced the extraordinary sensation of spontaneous transference of healing energy from one to the other.

A different aspect of healing involves the invocation of outside powers – sometimes those of religion or of the spirit world. Again, this is usually accomplished through the agency of a charismatic individual. But it may also be accomplished by prayer, through seance or by contact with a special shrine or sanctuary such as Lourdes.

There can be no doubt that this type of healing has worked on occasion – by whatever means.

The phenomenon of certain celebrated healers who produced extraordinary results again and again has never satisfactorily been explained away by sceptics. The fact that such cures cannot always be reproduced under laboratory conditions is not sufficient in itself to dismiss so much positive evidence. Indeed, one or two healers have also produced remarkable results in the laboratory – using animals, artificially cultured human cells and enzymes.

Psychic healing may well be resorted to where the patient lacks sufficient vitality to mobilise his or her self-healing power, and where doctors or other therapists can do little.

But the sufferer should not rely on such healing alone. Thorough medical diagnosis and advice must always be obtained first. Also there can be no reason why the healing process should not also be assisted by whichever other therapies are considered relevant to the particular condition.

Useful Address

British Society of Medical and Dental Hypnosis 15 Otley Old Road, Leeds LS16 6HN. Tel. 0532 613077

All members are qualified doctors or dentists and use hypnosis as part of conventional medical treatment.

Osteopathy and Chiropractic

Background

These therapies gained their initial impetus from the discovery that manipulation of the spine affects other parts of the body and may even be effective in the treatment of disease remote from the back.

The differences between osteopathy and chiropractic lie largely in their history and in their underlying theories. As actually practiced in this country today, their distinct ideologies and methods have tended to blur. Both are now greatly in demand – for back trouble in particular – but treatment of other ailments is also undertaken, especially by chiropractors.

History

Osteopathy was founded in 1874 by a physician, Andrew Taylor Still, as a result of his experience in the American Civil War. Andrew Still believed that much disease arose from faulty alignment of the spinal vertebrae which caused pressure on the arteries and impeded circulation of the blood, and that this can be cured by manipulation. He vehemently opposed orthodox medicine and, in turn, attracted hostility and derision.

Chiropractic is also American in origin. It was started in 1895 by David Daniel Palmer, a grocer and part-time osteopath and healer. Palmer achieved some spectacular cures for deafness and heart trouble by spinal manipulation. He then went on to formulate a theory which attributes the cause of disease to interference with the flow of nervous energy, arising from maladjustment of the spine.

The Position Today

Over the years, osteopathy outgrew Still's original notion of arterial pressure causing disease. Relaxation of this and of other parts of its earlier stance brought osteopathy very much closer to the medical profession. It is now regarded by doctors as a complementary therapy. A few of them practise as osteopaths and more have received some training in the application of this therapy.

Naturopaths frequently also qualify in osteopathy which, with chiropractic, forms an important part of many of their prescribed programmes of cure.

Osteopaths believe fully in a holistic approach to patients and their problems. However, because of their great popularity and the consequent pressure on their time, they now tend to concentrate on their own therapy and to refer the emotional and nutritional aspects of total cure to other specialists.

Chiropractic still maintains the basic beliefs of its founder, though in a less extreme form. These are, of course, contrary to the views of conventional medicine; and this has caused chiropractic to remain very much an alternative therapy.

American chiropractors often treat a general run of patients – especially in districts where conventional medical care is scarce. Then they act very much as family doctors.

In this country, chiropractors and osteopaths tend to specialise in back problems. The theory behind each therapy is not therefore of primary importance to the majority of patients who come to a therapist for the relief of back pain which conventional medicine can do little to help. For example, the author's wife – completely uninterested in the basis of chiropractic – found to her astonishment that several minutes of gentle manipulation by a chiropractor, encountered at a health farm to which she had resorted for diet and rest, permanently cured the chronic back pain she had been enduring for the previous ten years.

Diagnosis   Diagnosis starts with the case history and close observation of the patient's posture at rest and in movement. A more detailed examination then follows, involving the probing and palpating of the spinal region in particular, as well as close observation of what happens as the limbs are moved in various ways by the therapist.

An osteopath, to whom the case may well have been referred by a doctor or naturopath, may be content with all the information gathered by the two sources.

The chiropractor, on the other hand, is far more likely to have X-rays taken as well as a variety of other tests – blood, urine, orthopaedic and neurological – to build up the complete picture.

Treatment

Methods of manipulation used by practitioners of the two therapies once differed substantially – with osteopaths using the arms and legs for leverage on the joints and chiropractors working directly on the focus of trouble. Those distinctions have by now largely disappeared.

Arthritis and Rheumatism

Osteopathy is not often used on its own but more usually in conjunction with other therapies. It does not attempt a complete cure and makes few claims to be able to reverse degenerative joint damage that has already taken place. It is of value in preventing further deterioration. Inflammation and other distressing symptoms may be reduced with its aid and joint mobility much improved.

The first part of the process consists of a specialised massage of soft tissues in the affected area. The therapist's fingers probe the muscles, seeking out stresses and adhesions which are then eased. This relieves muscular tension on neighbouring joints and promotes the drainage of swollen regions with consequent lessening of stiffness and pain.

This is usually sufficient for the treatment of rheumatic complaints. Where arthritic joints are also involved, the therapist then proceeds to manipulate those joints in order to stretch adhesions and break down resistance to movement. This can be done either gradually or more abruptly.

The high velocity thrust method is the one for which osteopaths are best known. Usually applied to the spine and neighbouring joints, their forceful abrupt wrenches are followed by an alarming cracking sound. The process is usually painless; but when it does hurt, the therapist will explain that a sharp jolt to free a joint may be less painful in the long run than gentler but prolonged manipulation.

Setting theory aside, the practical approaches of both chiropractic and osteopathy to the treatment of rheumatic disease now differ by subtle degrees of emphasis rather than in substance.

The chiropractor may be more aware of the relief of nerve irritation as one aim of his technique. He may make more use of trigger or reflex points to achieve his purpose. He may tend to give more attention to the upper vertebrae than to the lower. But all this matters little to the patient on the therapy table. It is the end result that counts.

Soft tissue massage is used in chiropractic very much as in osteopathy. Manipulation of the joints is mostly carried out using the precise short sharp thrusts traditional to the therapy. But in recent years, chiropractors and osteopaths have borrowed much in the way of technique from each other, with mutual benefit.

Statistics

Chiropractic has received impressive confirmation of its value in the treatment of back pain in the United States. Figures released by no fewer that four separate State Workmen's Compensation Commissions show that claimants treated by chiropractors return to work much sooner than those under conventional medical care. Their treatment is far cheaper and they suffer less.

Professional Organisations

The British Chiropractic Association
   10 Greycoat Place London SW1P 1SB. Tel. 071 222 8866
This association runs a clinic and an information service. It maintains a register of qualified chiropractors, over 200 of whom are in practice in the U.K.

The General Council and Register of Osteopaths Ltd.
   56 London Street, Reading, Berks. RG1 4SQ.
Tel. 0734 576 585 This maintains a register of qualified osteopaths, of which over 800 are in practice in the U.K.

British Osteopathic Association
   8 Boston Place, London NW1. Telephone 071 262 5250.
Between fifty and one hundred of its members practise in the U.K. They are all qualified doctors as well as osteopaths.

Joint Mobilisation
(Spinal Mobilisation)

This technique, used by some physiotherapists, is based partly on the work of Geoffrey Maitland of Adelaide, Australia. It is fully described by Sarah Key in her book *Back in Action*, published by Century.

Sarah Key, who has successfully treated Prince Charles, claims that *thousands upon thousands* will testify that her methods work.

The underlying belief is that a stiff and painful spinal joint can be gradually eased by movement until it attains a new equilibrium. The more such a joint is made to move, the more it stretches and clears itself of its stiffness and pain. Though most often used on the complex joints of the spine, for backache, the principle and method apply equally to all joints.

The therapist first searches out the areas of stiffness in the spine by probing with the thumbs. Stiff joints are soon discovered, as they feel hard and unyielding to the touch and resist movement.

The next and most important step is to prise free the locked joint – not with the kind of sudden movement used in osteopathy, but more gently. Pressure is applied, usually through the therapist's thumbs, easily but relentlessly pushing and then releasing until movement is achieved.

Repeated treatment is reinforced by a series of specially designed exercises until the joint has regained sufficient strength to remain stable in its newly mobile condition.

Sarah Key's book is highly recommended for further reading. It clearly explains many back problems as well as describing her own method of treatment.

Massage and Rolfing

Remedial Massage

A good massage simultaneously relaxes the body and stimulates some of its functions. It also soothes the mind. The resulting feeling of well-being is of assistance in every kind of holistic treatment, whether conventional or alternative.

Massage is useful for sufferers from rheumatic disease, with one important proviso – it should not be applied in acute conditions during an active inflammatory phase of arthritis.

When properly employed, massage eases muscular tension and reduces emotional stress. It improves blood circulation and stimulates lymphatic drainage. Furthermore, it is pleasurable!

Swedish Massage, the most common form in present use, starts with a stroking motion to relax the body for what follows. Then comes the typical kneading, pinching and rolling of the deeper tissues. Specific tensions are dissolved by circular rubbing movements and stimulus is given by a combination of striking and chopping.

Rolfing

Rolfing, or Structural Integration, is a particularly intense system of massage, finally perfected in the 1960's by Dr Ida Rolf.

It is an extreme therapy, suitable for rheumatism and some chronic back pain, but not appropriate for the treatment of many kinds of arthritis.

The expressed aim of rolfing is to correct faulty posture. This relieves the strains to which the spinal column and its associated muscles and other tissues have become subjected, thus removing the cause of illness and chronic pain.

A typical course of treatment consists of ten one-hour sessions, during which the therapist's body weight is used to press very deeply into the patient. The connective tissues, on which posture depends, are first systematically loosened by this searching treatment and then realigned.

From all accounts, rolfing is a drastic and painful experience – physically and emotionally. It is claimed to be very effective in resolving harmful muscular and mental stresses.

Rolfing is taught only in the United States of America. *The Rolf Institute*, P.O.Box 1868, Boulder, Colorado 80302, U.S.A., maintains an international register of qualified practitioners.

Alexander Technique

History

F.M. Alexander had just started to earn his living as an actor in Australia when he unaccountably started to lose his voice in the middle of Shakespeare recitals. Doctors could do nothing to help.

Alexander slowly began to realise that the basic fault lay in his tendency to stiffen his neck and pull his head back and down when declaiming. In the process of slowly ridding himself of this disabling habit, he noticed that some of his negative personality traits – such as a foul temper – also improved.

Alexander died in 1955 at the age of eighty-six, having devoted his life to developing the ideas and method that now bear his name. He treated many famous people and himself became a cult figure.

Recent interest in alternative therapies of all kinds has helped to spread public awareness of the Alexander Technique, which is now taught widely both in the United Kingdom and in America.

Theory

Alexander believed that the spine, to which every organ of the body is in some way connected, is the key to physical and mental health.

Unlike many naturopaths, he maintained that the spine is well-designed and fully suited to its purpose. Modern man, having lost his instinctive awareness of how the body functions, soon acquires bad habits of posture and in the use of muscles. This affects body and mind, one being fully dependent on the other.

Alexander Technique involves learning a series of physical movements designed to correct bad posture, bring the body back into correct alignment and help it to function efficiently. It relies on the assumption that bad habits are not instinctive; and that they can be unlearned and then replaced by better ones.

Another basic belief is that body, mind and emotions all act together and cannot be separated, one from the other. Those who are mentally troubled or stressed show this in their body language. It is only through correcting the body that these strains too can be relieved.

Therapy

Alexander Technique is not a self-help therapy and definitely requires lessons from a skilled teacher, on a one-to-one basis.

Full awareness of the body, in repose and in motion, is taught with the aim of achieving perfect balance and poise.

Bad habits are gradually unlearned. Correct posture and muscle use is substituted, with emphasis on the head and neck. A good illustration of the ideal posture is to think of the top of the head being attached to an invisible cord which is gently being pulled upwards towards the sky. This would tend to lengthen the spine, simultaneously bringing body, neck and head into true alignment.

Arthritis and Rheumatism

By releasing muscular tension, and stopping further damage from bad posture, the body is enabled to start on its self-healing process.

Soft tissue complaints and all kinds of back pain and arthritis are therefore high on the list of conditions claimed to benefit from application of the Alexander Technique.

The Technique also acts powerfully to relieve mental stress – again to the benefit of sufferers from arthritis, rheumatism, asthma, migraine and depression.

Professional Body

The Society of Teachers of the Alexander Technique
London House, 266 Fulham Road, London SW10 9EL.
Telephone 071 351 0828.

There are roughly 300 members in practice in the U.K.

Feldenkrais

Background Moshe Feldenkrais was an Israeli scientist and judo master who died in 1984. Refusing uncertain surgery for an old knee injury which threatened to disable him, Feldenkrais began to realise how the way he moved his knee contributed to the pain he was experiencing. He then went on to study the part played by the knee in the movement of his whole body – and eventually cured himself by applying what he had discovered.

Like Alexander before him, Feldenkrais developed a sophisticated series of exercises to promote awareness of body movement, with particular emphasis on proper use of the muscles. The brain is, in effect, programmed to promote maximum efficiency in both body and mind.

Uses Feldenkrais himself built up a considerable reputation for his treatment of patients with cerebral palsy. His technique is also particularly recommended for people with neuromuscular trouble and chronic pain for which doctors can do little. It is only mentioned briefly here because of the scarcity of practitioners in this country.

Though teachers of the Feldenkrais method make no claim to be able to cure arthritis, they do make sufferers feel better, move more easily and experience less pain. Reduction in strain on arthritic joints will help to inhibit further damage and may stimulate healing.

As flare-ups of rheumatoid arthritis are often related to mental stress, it is believed that the relaxation and sense of well-being resulting from the application of this technique can reduce the severity and even the frequency of such crises.

Availability Though very popular in the United States of America, there are few teachers of Feldenkrais in the U.K.

Information may be obtained from *The Feldenkrais Guild* P.O. Box 370, London N10 3XA.

Part Five

Sensitivity Therapy

Introduction

What is here described as Sensitivity Therapy has been left to the end of the book, and given a special part of its own, for two very good reasons.

The first is that it belongs neither with conventional medicine nor with the alternative therapies.

It is not an alternative therapy because it relies on no special theories that cannot be explained or demonstrated by conventional means. Its methods are wholly scientific, being those of experiment and observation.

On the other hand, it has not yet been embraced by the medical profession which has generally displayed little interest, even in published results of clinical trials.

The second reason for giving the subject a part of its own in this book is that it seems to offer exciting new prospects on the frontier of attempts to understand arthritis and find a cure.

Food Sensitivity

It is almost an article of faith for some nature therapists to believe that, as man has been consuming grains and dairy foods for only the past ten thousand or so years of his long history, an abnormal sensitivity to them, as well as to over-refined products such as sugar and unnatural ones like chemical preservatives, is a likely cause of arthritis and other chronic ailments. However, such belief is not in any way central to the many extraordinary claims that abstention from certain foodstuffs has effected dramatic improvement in bad cases of rheumatoid arthritis.

Libraries and bookshops contain many volumes written by people who recovered from crippling disease by eliminating certain foods from their diets. Many tried to start eating those foods again, on a selective basis, only to find that their symptoms returned.

A large number of popular books have been written on diet as a cure for arthritis. One of the ones readily available when this survey was being prepared is by Giraud W. Campbell and published by Thorsons. It is entitled *A Doctor's Proven New Home Cure for Arthritis.*

In it, the author describes in detail a seven-day programme for relieving the symptoms of osteo or rheumatoid arthritis and confidently promises success for his method. It begins with a twenty-four hour fast and continues with only fresh raw food and vegetables. Other selected foods are introduced later as the symptoms diminish. Campbell's other recommendations include heavy emphasis on elimination through the bowels, osteopathic manipulation, neuromuscular stimulation, selected herbs and supplements and gentle exercise. A strict diet is the key; and this must be continued indefinitely if symptoms are not to recur.

In its essentials, Campell's method is very similar to those of Nurse Hills, Anna Scott and Leon Chaitow, described in Part Four of this book, as well as to those of many others. It is claimed that thousands of sufferers worldwide have benefited from this kind of dietary exclusion therapy. All these people certainly are not lying – and this is demonstrated by the grudging admission by the medical profession that *there may be something in it* as, inexplicably, the treatment does work in at least a few cases.

Perhaps the main reason why this type of treatment has not gained wider acceptance is that it may succeed only in a small number of cases. Just how small is a matter of keen controversy. But this suggests that sensitivity to a few foods really is too simple an explanation to be accepted as the cause of arthritis.

Allergy

Source

The source of much of the information in this section is a book entitled *Arthritis – The Allergy Connection,* written by Dr John Mansfield and published by Thorsons. This is highly recommended for further reading.

Environmental Control Clinics

These are special purpose-built units, guaranteed free from all substances that could cause allergic reactions. Mansfield observes that a very large majority of arthritis sufferers, who undertake to fast for several days within such a unit, improve spectacularly during that time.

A likely conclusion is that arthritis must either be caused or at the very least be seriously aggravated by the food or other environmental factors left outside the units.

The results also seem to dispose of the theory that rheumatoid arthritis is caused by auto-immunity – that is, by the body reacting against itself.

A problem arises, though, in explaining why about ten per cent of patients show no improvement when fasting in the allergy-free environment. Dr. Mansfield explains that some are allergic to organisms (thrush) within their own bowels, brought into the unit with them; and that the remainder have had their immune systems so damaged by prolonged drug-taking that they have become incapable of responding.

The Basic Theory

This is that nearly all forms of arthritis are related to intolerance to certain environmental factors – which include foodstuffs, chemicals, polluted air, house dust, and air-born moulds.

Arthritis may therefore be treated by determining and then removing its cause, rather than by attempting merely to suppress its symptoms as in more orthodox medicine.

Detection of the responsible allergens may be simple or complex; but it can be done.

If allergens thus identified can be avoided in daily life, all well and good. If this is just too difficult, several lengthy techniques are available to de-sensitise the sufferer to enable him or her to tolerate most of such substances.

The Theory in More Detail

It seems that food sensitivities or allergies are far more complex than originally supposed. They can involve a large number of foods at the same time and be complicated by reaction to chemicals introduced into the food chain by the use of fertilisers, pesticides and preservatives. Sensitivity to the chlorine in tap water, for example, is quoted by Dr. Mansfield as an important factor in the cure of one of his own patients.

To make matters worse, people may also to some extent be addicted to those foods to which they are most sensitive. Thus, allergic reaction is masked by withdrawal symptoms when the offending foods are removed from the diet, and by a temporary boost when they are restored.

It has been found that sufferers from arthritis may also be reacting to various substances which are inhaled during the course of their daily lives. House dust and dust mites, natural (North Sea) gas and the common air-born moulds are prime examples. This may explain why arthritics are specially sensitive to the onset of thunderstorms, for that is a time when the mould count is often unusually high.

Identification

Only the simplest food allergies can be tackled successfully on a do-it-yourself basis. Most other cases will need specialised help to disentangle the complex web of cause and effect; and this may be another reason why this new approach to arthritis has not yet received the attention it deserves.

Allergy diagnosis and treatment may be obtained at any one of about a dozen out-patient clinics in this country. Advice on their locations and suitability may be obtained from *Action Against Allergy*, a voluntary organisation working in this field. Its address is 24 High Street, Hampton Hill, Middlesex TW12 1PD.

At such clinics, elimination diets will be tried as well as a new and most effective method of skin testing, far superior to the type in general use. Answers to precisely what troubles most patients will be found.

A few really complicated cases, though, will require more rigorous in-patient investigation to produce the right answers.

They can be tackled only at one of the two environmental control units currently operating in this country – *The Airedale Allergy Centre,* Keighley, Yorkshire and *The Breakespeare Hospital,* King's Langley, Hertfordshire.

As described earlier, these consist of special units, maintained free from all known allergens. In them, patients fast for several days during which their symptoms disappear or are much improved. Tests are then carried out, one by one, with selected organically produced foods and with other substances administered by inhalation.

Treatment

Once food and environmental sensitivities have been identified, diets can be planned to avoid offending foods and chemicals. Steps can also be taken to avoid some environmental hazards. If, for example, natural gas is a problem, domestic cooking can be changed from gas to electric and the gas boiler can be resited in an outside cupboard.

Neutralisation Therapy

In cases of real difficulty, most but not quite all allergies can be overcome by a method known as provocative neutralisation therapy. This is far more effective and much safer that the old method of desensitisation, which involves injecting the patient with large and increasing doses of the offending substance.

Provocative neutralisation therapy is based on a discovery made by an American doctor in 1957. He found that he could induce symptoms of asthma in his wife (who suffered badly from asthma) by injecting her with a specific dose of a particular substance to which she was sensitive. He also discovered that her symptoms would disappear completely within minutes after he had injected her with another, much smaller, specific dose of the same substance. Doses that differed from the specific ones had little effect. This is, of course, a curious echo of the homeopathic principle described in Part Four of this book.

Doses are injected into the skin and have to be taken regularly every two days. Modern *automatic* insulin syringes – painless, easy to use and disposable – are recommended to enable patients to administer the small injections themselves with minimum effort.

Treatment has to continue for about two years for the neutralisation to become permanent. Re-testing will have to be carried out at least once in that period, as the amount of the required neutralising dose has been found to change during the course of treatment.

The Intestinal Tract

Another small but important factor identified by Dr. Mansfield in arthritis treatment is intestinal candidiasis or thrush as it is commonly called. Candida is a yeast-like organism which inhabits the intestinal tract and is usually harmless.

However, the prolonged use of broad-spectrum antibiotics or steroids can disturb the balance and enable the thrush to multiply alarmingly and produce various unpleasant symptoms.

When this happens, fungi penetrate the lining of the intestines, creating a leaky condition in which partly digested substances can penetrate back into the body. (Note the echo of naturopathic theory.) The fungi also release a very large number of chemical substances, against which the body has to provide resistance.

It is thought that some of the arthritis sufferers, who respond negatively to food and environmental sensitivity tests, are in fact reacting against allergens produced within their own intestines; and several stubborn cases have been cleared up on that basis.

Thrush can be treated by special diets and by courses of anti-fungal medicines.

Epilogue

A Personal View

In writing this book, its author had two main aims in view. The first was to persuade sufferers from rheumatic disease that relief from its worst symptoms, if not a cure, was in their own hands; and that they should not delay in engaging in this most worthwhile struggle. The second was to present a detached and balanced survey of the claims made by the advocates of each of the many kinds of therapy – both orthodox medical and alternative – for their respective systems.

The author approached his task with a relatively open mind, having no fixed prior views on arthritis treatment. However, a conventional scientific training and professional life may have introduced some subconscious bias in which aromatherapy, for example, could not be taken quite as seriously as a modern *wonder* drug as the basis of treatment.

Research on the ideas underlying many of the so-called alternative therapies, and a cool assessment of what conventional treatment has to offer, caused the writer to review some of his own previously held concepts on science, health and disease. Though not allowing this to influence the balance of the text, some of what he concluded is set out in this brief epilogue.

The first thought, hardly original, is that scientists at many stages of human history have decided they had the key to understanding natural phenomena. One only has to look at modern theories of the origins and composition of the universe, of matter and energy, to see how rapidly old certainties have recently dissolved. Natural scientists have been wrong more often than right. It is arrogant to close one's mind to forms of intuitive understanding, even if these cannot be expressed in acceptable modern terms.

A simple example is that of the water diviner. Water divining certainly works and is used by many hard-headed business organisations – but no one knows why it works and no conventional scientific explanation seems possible.

The intuitive concept that a human being is a single entity – body, mind and spirit – is at the back of most alternative systems of medicine, whether ancient Chinese or modern American. So too is the idea that an arthritic joint, for example, should not only be tackled in isolation, as one would repair or change a defective machine part, but should be considered also as a symptom of a deeper malaise affecting the whole person.

An antibiotic, for example, efficiently kills all the germs but leaves the basic cause – why the germs were able to invade the body so successfully – untreated. The antibiotic is a quick and most welcome remedy. But the possibility that the underlying cause may then be driven deeper underground, to manifest itself in another and possibly more serious illness later, is disturbing.

There can be no doubt that the human body possesses the mysterious power of constantly being able to renew its own living cells and also of healing itself from most injuries and diseases. Any means of strengthening this ability of self-healing must therefore make good sense.

Drugs can save lives and provide rapid relief. When used to excess they are potentially more dangerous than the diseases they are used to treat. A major source of funds used in medical research is provided by drug companies, eager both to benefit humanity and, very properly, to earn profits for themselves. Unfortunately there seems little money available for the research so badly needed on alternative medicine.

Little of what has been written above would be questioned by any thinking doctor. But as medicine has to be practised in today's conditions, few doctors have the time to be able to take such ideas to their logical conclusions. Alternative therapists, on the other hand, have both the time and the urge to transform such beliefs into practical action.

What then would the author do himself if faced with the onset of a chronic, incurable disease such as arthritis? First, he would obtain the best medical diagnosis and advice at the earliest possible moment. He would remain under the general care of an open-minded and sympathetic doctor. He would resort to surgery if indicated, but only after thorough investigation of alternatives and the likely outcome.

If infection or excruciating pain was involved, the author would most probably not be able to resist the temptation of a quick fix, using antibiotics and pain-killing drugs.

However, the next stage would certainly be to try out the allergy therapy described in Part Five of this book.

If that failed, he would get his GP to refer him to the best hospital rheumatology outpatients' clinic available locally to see what conventional management is on offer. In conjunction with that, he would most probably experiment with one of the major forms of alternative therapy outlined in Part Four of the book. Which therapy would depend on further study and what was available in his neighbourhood. A dedicated therapist with a record of success would be a prime requirement.

An all-out onslaught would be planned, employing one or more subsidiary disciplines in addition to the principal one. Homeopathy, acupuncture, nutrition, chiropractic or osteopathy would certainly qualify for inclusion if appropriate. Some self-help methods, including relaxation technique, would be considered, as would a form of psychotherapy if needed. The total care programme offered by the *Arthritic Association* (page 73 above) sounds attractive and would be investigated in depth.

The only possible alternative to this fringe activity would be the kind of conventional but comprehensive programme described in Part Three of this book. This is offered to patients by the Stanford Arthritis Centre of California; but such total care and guidance is not always available.

To summarise, the author's advice is never to accept as inevitable a chronic illness such as arthritis, but to engage fully in a determined struggle to overcome it by one way or another. Efforts should be made to keep the use of drugs to the minimum by the use of conventional or alternative therapy. An open mind should be brought to the question of trying treatments based on the alternative view of health and disease, for it is claimed that many thousands of people have benefited from such an approach. If the disease then goes into natural remission of its own accord, and not because of the efforts made, the activity has been wasted – but in such circumstances, will that really matter?

Index